BREATHE, CHILL

A Handy Book of Games and Techniques Introducing Breathing, Meditation and Relaxation to Kids and Teens

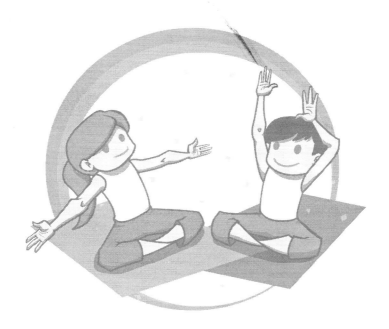

Lisa Roberts RYT, RCYT

Cover Image and Illustration: Amrit Tigga

Cover Design and Typesetting: Art Fact India

Library of Congress Control Number: 2014902633

ISBN: 1495314693
ISBN-13: 978-1495314698

DEDICATION

Breathe, Chill *is warmly dedicated to my favorite high school teacher, Dr. Arthur Mowle. And all teachers who are brave enough to move beyond curriculum, imparting valuable life-skills with humor, wisdom and sensitivity.*

Praise for *Breathe, Chill*

"A must read for parents, healthcare providers, day care workers, teachers, or any one that has an opportunity to be with children and teens; Breathe, Chill *provides fun and educational activities that can be taught to all ages, in any setting. Roberts' real life experiences combined with her intellect, compassion for children/teens, and desire to teach creates a beneficial experience for all."*

Jill Malan, Manager Child Life Services, St. Louis Children's Hospital

"Therapists, counselors, teachers and other professionals who want to provide children and youth with skills in self-regulation, relaxation and mindfulness should use this book. The easy-to-follow directions and diagrams make yoga and meditation accessible in any setting."

Beth Reese, LPC, Psychotherapist

"With a colorful repertoire of engaging exercises, Roberts' how-to book will promote wellness in our most precious resource: our young people."

Katherine Van Uum, Philosopher, Girl Scout Leader, Mother

"The techniques of proper breathing and relaxation are cleverly adapted to assist leaders in guiding children in these wonderful exercises. Children who are taught these exercises in the fun methods described will undoubtedly benefit from them. Kudos on an excellent teaching guide for parents, teachers, and anyone who works with children!"

Melissa E. Chatfield, RN, PhD

"The science backs up this much needed prescription for breathing deeply and deliberately. Roberts makes the serious business of mindful, meditation techniques accessible and fun. Responsible parents should buy this book before resorting to behavior modification prescription medications for their children. Say no to drugs and say yes to breathing and yoga."

Richard A. Masla, Founder and Director Ayurveda Health Retreat, Alachua, FL.

*"*Breathe, Chill *contains 'any age'- friendly techniques for gaining knowledge and experience with breath, movement and mindfulness activities. Roberts has brilliantly organized each activity ensuring accessibility of use. This is a great resource for anyone who wishes to empower children to connect to their inner wisdom, strength and resilience. She teaches life long skills that will help children navigate through every age. As a pediatric occupational therapist, these activities are a fabulous adjunct to traditional therapy for they honor the child where they are on the path of their life while building inner resources and awareness to heal and connect. This will certainly be a treasure for parents, teachers, yoga practitioners and therapists."*

Allison Morgan, MA, OTR, RYT
Pediatric Occupational Therapist, Children's Yoga Instructor and Founder, Zensational Kids

"Breathe, Chill *offers insight to the best yoga has to offer – how to relax and just breathe. Presented in layman's terms, it's easy and accessible to anyone who wants to learn the art of relaxation. Plus, it's just plain fun!*"

Jennifer Grant, Writer, Yoga Instructor

"Breathe, Chill *provides ways to build awareness of your body and breathing and how to use them beneficially. Stress is normal, but we do not always cope with it in a positive way.* Breathe, Chill *teaches kids, teens, and adults easy to understand methods to be proactive with stress and incorporate relaxation into their day.*"

Anne Rosenberg, B.S. Special Education
(Academic Assistance/Tutorial Support Services)

"*Learn. Practice. Breathe. Chill. What a perfect mantra for* Breathe, Chill. *I wish I had this book in my classroom when I taught 4th grade and we took daily yoga breaks.* Breathe, Chill *is broken down perfectly, allowing anyone to guide others (or themselves) through these exercises: What is it? How does it help me? How do I do it? - These are questions that I am asked naturally by my toddler daily. Most activities can be adapted to accommodate the needs of little ones who often need re-centering and calming. A great alternative to taking a "time out", these activities actually let you take a break and re-center in a fun way without feeling like you are being punished. I can't wait to watch my children grow, change, and find new connections and experiences as they practice these exercises!*"

Cathy Hilburg, Elementary Teacher, Mother of Two

"Breathe, Chill *is a wonderful resource book for any parent, teacher, or professional who works with or has children. The book provides a wealth of well-balanced exercises in an easy to read layout. I found the "what", "why", "how" format and clever illustrations very clear and easy to follow. I look forward to trying some of these 'fun' techniques myself!*"

Carol Pomerantz, Child Educator and Private Piano Instructor

"*We live in a very fast paced culture. Our modern way of living affects our children and who they will become as the next generation of leaders & teachers. Roberts simply and expertly explains techniques specifically designed for children to unplug and TUNE IN! This is the stuff that they should be learning in school. This book is a wonderful and practical tool for the modern child.*"

Syama Masla, Co-Founder Stanton Street Yoga, NYC and Kaivalya Retreats

Table of Contents

Acknowledgements

First of all, I would like to thank Amrit Tigga for his excellent illustrations, not only did he skillfully translate my mediocre stick figure sketches into the fabulous artwork gracing the pages of this book, but he did so with a sense of humor and compassion.

This book would not be possible had the ancient wisdom of yoga not been passed along from teacher to student, generation to generation, for over five thousand years. Yogic wisdom has stretched its way to a broader audience as those who practice experience its many benefits and feel compelled to share it.

I would like to thank all of my teachers – not only those who taught the courses where I gained my qualifications, but those who teach the yoga classes I attend as a student. I am always learning, experiencing different teachers and studios in different cities around the world, and they all offer something – a new insight or simple instruction that not only benefits my personal yoga practice, but the students I teach.

Which leads me to the best teachers of all, my students! Each class brings a fresh opportunity to grow and learn, for the student and the teacher – it brings me so much joy to work with the children, teens and adults who allow me the honor of sharing the magic of yoga, breathing and meditation with them.

The patients I have worked with, who have trusted me to share their space during what can be a very personal and stressful period, approaching yoga, breath work and meditation techniques with a sense of curiosity, openness and willingness to learn. These valuable experiences have given me the opportunity to develop as a teacher and provided the inspiration for this book.

Most importantly, I am deeply grateful for my greatest breath of fresh air, my husband Michael. An amazing and beloved husband and friend, he is also an excellent sounding board, proofreader, coach, and personal stylist (with enviable fashion sense!). A resistant yogi, Michael is by far the greatest teacher I have experienced, challenging me to find ways to serve up the wisdom of yoga in a way that appeals to, and benefits, all – regardless of culture, gender, age, or interest in yoga. You really do not have to "yoga" to yoga, unless, of course, you want to.

A Note From the Author

In 1988 my parents removed me from the public high school I had been attending and enrolled me in a private co-ed catholic school. I was terribly nervous, the "new girl" rarely fared well at my previous school; an easy target for the mean kids, any newbie was openly ridiculed and harassed. Trepidations also arose due the fact that I was not catholic, and the new school included an almost daily compulsory religious studies class. My sixteen-year-old self bristled at the notion of having a religion I knew nothing about shoved down my throat on a daily basis. Two things happened when I arrived at my new school that year: I was welcomed with warmth by my fellow students, and I met Dr. Arthur Mowle, the school psychologist who also happened to be my religious studies teacher.

Doc Mowle, as many of the students fondly called him, and I did not form any special student/teacher bond while I was at school, in fact I was so shy and quiet I doubt I left a lasting impression on any of my teachers. I LOVED his classes, yet I never talked about this teacher to my friends or family, nor referred to him as my favorite and most impactful teacher…. until many years later when the wisdom he subtly laced his classes with bubbled to the surface of my consciousness.

Fast forward to 2001, recovering from a nephrectomy following a kidney cancer diagnosis, I decided to make use of my newly found spare time and embark on Vipassana studies – something I had been dying to do since being introduced to Buddhism during a five year stint living in Asia in my early twenties.

I signed up for a 10-day silent retreat to study this style of meditation derived from Buddhism. Frustrated and unable to quiet my mind one afternoon, I stormed out of the meditation hall and took myself on a long walk around the perimeter of the property hoping to achieve success practicing walking meditation. As I walked I told myself, "Look at the sky", "Look at the trees", "Notice each branch"…. And BOOM! Lightening struck!

While this was no life altering, earth shattering type of enlightenment, it certainly was an epiphany. "Oh my gosh," I thought to myself, "this is what Doc Mowle was teaching us all those years ago." I smiled as I came to the realization that my eleventh-grade religious studies teacher – the very class I feared most before starting at my new school – had surreptitiously taught his students present moment awareness and walking meditation skills.

Thinking back to his class, at the age of 29, thirteen years removed from my hideous bottle green uniform and black lace-up shoes, I understood everything he had given me in that moment – rich, valuable life lessons disguised as afternoon walks, and lively discussions about life, death, and everything in between.

In lieu of bible studies, Doc Mowle raised topics – sometimes controversial— and then opened the class to discussion. Nobody was right, nobody was wrong, and each student had the opportunity to speak his or her mind – differing opinions, thoughts and ideas were proffered in a safe environment without judgment. From these discussions we learned to value and respect one another as human beings, opening our minds to possibility of differing opinions and varying points of view without feeling the need to alter our own.

Our afternoon strolls—the ones where my sixteen-year old self thought, "Woohoo, I am getting out of school for 45 minutes! —taught us to be aware of our surroundings and to be fully present, "Look at the sky," "Look at the trees,"... notice the details. Be here. Be. Finally, I understood *why* I had loved Doc Mowle's class.

I was, quite simply, blown away by the foundation that had been laid by one teacher in one class thirteen years prior. Since that day, I never shut up about Doc Mowle, singing his praises to anybody who would listen.

In 2011, I listened as I raved how wonderful he was to a lunch companion and stopped myself mid-sentence, embarrassed that I never bothered to thank him, I vowed to do so as soon as I returned home that afternoon. A few short emails to my old school, then the school Doc had transferred to long ago (and since retired from) and voila! I was in touch with Doc Mowle.

Of course, the school had asked his permission before sharing his information with me and I was embarrassed once more when Doc Mowle reached out to me before I had a chance to send him my thank you note. Once I did express my gratitude and interpretation of his classes, he confirmed that I was correct. He had, over the years, caught some criticism for his methods, yet he remained steadfast – his many years of teaching experience had proven this was the right approach. His place, he told me, was not to tell his students who or what God was, or where to find God, but to guide them to find their own God in their own unique situation.

How does this story relate to the book I have written? As a yoga teacher and yoga therapist I continually meet people who feel a little apprehensive – not unlike myself at sixteen heading off to catholic school—that yoga, breathing exercises and/or meditation are a form of religion, and that practicing may oppose the faith they are committed to. *Absolutely not!* Yoga, in my opinion, is simply breathing, and through this connection to breath many find a connection to their true self, and wherever that leads is a personal journey.

Teaching—any subject—is both an honor and a responsibility that should be taken seriously. Deeply influenced by my high school religious studies teacher, I make a point of not bringing anything remotely religious, or my own personal beliefs, into the classes I teach. The physical and mental benefits of yoga and meditation are what inspired me to practice, and, ultimately to teach. This is what I enjoy sharing with others, guiding them to explore and embrace their minds and bodies with curiosity, wonder and acceptance. Discovering how the mind and body work independently, together, and how they can work for the individual.

Through my work in pediatric hospitals, teaching patients experiencing extreme pain episodes, I created easy to follow handouts explaining the breath and meditation exercises from their weekly yoga sessions to allow them to continue practicing on their own. Intentionally shifting the focus away from their illness, I teach them how to use the techniques in every day situations, such as prior to a test or exam, allowing the children to make the connection that these techniques may also be helpful for pain control, or during uncomfortable medical procedures, to help them relax, giving them a sense of empowerment in the process. The handouts have proven to be immensely popular with patients, parents and staff. This book is a compilation of these handouts.

The intention of this book is to enable anybody working with children—regardless of their yoga experience—the ability to share the benefits of breathing and meditation techniques with the children in their lives. Working with children, we all share the common goal of enriching their lives and providing a solid, stable foundation to build happy, successful and healthy futures. Please use this book as a guide, share the exercises with the children in your life and you will be providing them with valuable tools and coping skills that they can access within themselves anywhere, any time, throughout life. Together we can make a difference.

Lisa Roberts RYT, RCYT

Disclaimer

The material in this book is provided for informational purposes only and may not be construed as medical advice or instruction. Proper discretion should be used, in conjunction with consultation with healthcare professionals, before undertaking any of the exercises and techniques described in this book.

Introduction

Breathe, Chill – *A Handy Book of Games and Techniques Introducing Breathing, Meditation and Relaxation to Kids and Teens*

The physical and mental health benefits of practicing proper breathing techniques has been well documented in adults, and taking time out for a little R&R or short meditation break has been shown to reduce stress and increase productivity. Well, it is no different for kids! And with the over stimulated lifestyles they lead, it could be just what the doctor ordered.

Kids today are more stressed than ever before. Loaded with schoolwork, extra curricular activities, responsibilities and expectations, they experience physical stress from using computers and carrying heavy backpacks, as well as psychological stress from bullying and peer pressure. Technological advancements have introduced stressors into the lives of modern children that previous generations did not experience. Cyber-bullying is a big issue that has received a lot of attention in the media, but the need to always be connected along with the demand for instant gratification also grossly impacts our children's stress levels.

Invariably running in overdrive, they are distracted, unable to focus, and unequipped to cope when things do not go their way or when faced with challenging or stressful situations. Being constantly wired or in "go" mode is not a healthy state for anybody, and kids especially need to rest their minds and bodies, yet many children do not know how to slow things down, or relax.

Wouldn't it be great to equip our children with simple yet valuable life-skills they can access any time and anywhere to help them cope with the multiple stressors they endure? Providing them with the tools, knowledge and ability to calm, center, concentrate, and respond to stressful or difficult situations in a healthy and positive manner.

The MANY additional benefits of practicing breathing and meditation techniques extend beyond controlling stress: the practice of simple, proper breathing increases oxygen levels, improves blood circulation, improves posture, enhances mental clarity and the ability to focus, elevates mood states, and aids in pain control. Sounds extremely beneficial—*and necessary*—but how do you convey this to kids?

Most kids, when told that something is good for them, shy away from it. Not that they necessarily gravitate toward things that are bad for them, but "good" simply does not sound like "fun" to a kid. Can breathing and meditation techniques be engaging and fun for kids? Of course they can! Children do not need to sit in lotus posture chanting "ohm" or endure boring lectures about the advantages of taking slow, deep, diaphragmatic breaths–*and many children won't*—to benefit from, or learn, breathing and meditation techniques.

Like disguising broccoli in chocolate sauce, *Breathe, Chill– A Handy Book of Games and Techniques Introducing Breathing, Meditation and Relaxation to Kids and Teens* presents seventy fun breathing, meditation, and relaxation exercises and activities adapted for children of all ages.

Demonstrating that breath work and meditation can make them feel GREAT, some of the exercises offer an outlet for tension or stress, while others stealthily teach deep breathing skills, present moment awareness and relaxation … but, sshh, don't tell them it's good for them!

Breathe Chill is a practical resource for parents or anybody working with children of all ages. Divided into three sections – *Breath Play, Breathing Techniques*, and *Relaxation and Meditation Techniques* – each exercise is presented in a fun yet factual, kid-friendly language and is broken down in the same simple format: *What is it? How does it help me? How do I do it?* Adapted from traditional meditation, yoga nidra and pranayama techniques, ancient wisdom is served in a manner that is accessible to all, regardless of age, yoga or meditation experience, religious background, or spiritual beliefs.

Kids are able to put these techniques to use immediately – before a test, exam or presentation, or when dealing with interpersonal issues, such as stress resulting from bullying. Teachers can use these techniques to harness or release excess energy when a class becomes restless, and by encouraging students to explore how they feel after completing any of the exercises presented in this book, kids begin to recognize the many areas in their lives where these skills can be applied, life-skills that will carry them well into adulthood.

Beyond the classroom, the proven techniques presented in *Breath, Chill* are useful for anybody working with children. Written by Lisa Roberts, a certified Children's Yoga Therapist, Registered Yoga Teacher and Registered Children's Yoga Teacher, these exercises have been successfully shared with patients experiencing extreme pain episodes and stress from extended hospital stays. The simplicity and accessibility of these exercises allow nurses, child-life staff, social workers and parents, as well as the patients themselves, to continue working with the exercises long after their weekly yoga sessions with the author.

Enriching the lives of children everywhere, giving them the tools necessary to become happy, content and balanced individuals, is the common goal we share when working with children. If you work with children, or have children in your life, THIS BOOK IS FOR YOU… *and for them.*

Guidelines and Posture Tips

Teacher Guidelines

How to Use This Book:

Breathe, Chill is divided into three distinct sections – *Breath Play, Breathing Techniques,* and *Relaxation and Meditation Techniques.* A basic posture guide provides suggestions for seated, standing and supine postures to practice the games and techniques. When introducing breathing or relaxation techniques to kids, *Breath Play* is a great place to begin. Exploring the breath, and how it works within their own bodies, through play helps kids to develop the basic breath stabilization and control skills needed to practice some of the techniques in *Breathing Techniques* and *Relaxation and Meditation Techniques.*

Each technique is presented in a super simple, kid-friendly format – *What is it? How does it help me? How do I do it?* This format makes it very easy to locate the right technique for any situation – be it pain control, letting off steam, deep relaxation, or focusing a class before a lecture or test.

If props are needed they will be listed before the *"how to"* directions, along with suggestions for alternative props should you not have access to those suggested. The most important instruction for using this book is to jump right in and try all of the exercises, have fun with them, and find what works best for the children in your life.

Working With Younger Children:

Young kids can be overzealous when first learning breathing techniques. Be wary of this when working with younger children and encourage them to develop stable and controlled breathing patterns. This can be achieved by introducing *Breath Play* games first, practicing for short periods with breaks of normal breathing in between.

Once the children become comfortable with the games and display signs of developing control, slowly begin to introduce some of the techniques in *Breathing Techniques.* Most of the techniques in *Relaxation and Meditation Techniques* can be shared with young children immediately, without the need to work on breath control first.

The beauty of these exercises is that you do not need to explain why you are doing them, simply jump right in and guide younger children by practicing with them. Play, make it fun, and they will benefit! End each practice with an open discussion – explore and acknowledge any differences noticed in the way they breathed and how it made them feel.

Younger children may not make a conscious connection between the breath and their minds or bodies, yet subliminally they will come to understand that the way they breathe while playing the games or practicing the exercises helps them to feel better and more relaxed.

Working With Older Children and Teens:

Older children are curious to learn what each technique is and how it specifically helps them – the simple format the techniques are presented in allow for easy explanation and a handy way to share the information as a handout they can keep and refer back to any time they need it. Encourage an open discussion post practice to explore and acknowledge any differences noticed in the way they breathed and how that made them feel. Let them make the connections and encourage them to think about where they can apply these skills and practices in their lives.

While it may elicit some moans and groans, it is very important to have the kids disconnect from their electronic devices. Switch off all cell-phones and gadgets and put them aside before beginning. In extreme cases, such as a hospitalized patient who may need to keep their phone on so family can reach them, the phone may be switched to vibrate mode and kept near the child. Be judicious and be sure to convey the benefits of disconnecting to your students.

Cautions:

- The breath should never be forced. Even exercises where deep breathing is encouraged – it should feel natural, with steady and evenly controlled breaths. If the breath becomes choppy or strained, stop practicing immediately and return to normal breathing.
- Slowly increase the number of rounds and/or practice time for each exercise incrementally and approach each practice anew. No matter how long you practiced during a previous session, always begin slowly and build up to your comfort level.
- Short breaks to breathe normally are encouraged, especially when first working with breathing techniques.
- Correct posture is vital – it creates the space in the body needed to access the complete breathing system and allows one to be more comfortable while practicing. General posture will also improve, positively impacting the skeletal, muscular, digestive, and circulatory systems and improving self-esteem.

Handy-Dandy Tips:

- Music can be incorporated to add to the ambience and encourage deeper levels of relaxation. Ambient music can be found on iTunes, or CD's may be purchased at stores such as Target, Walmart, or music and health stores.
- Set the mood for relaxation by reducing harsh light and drawing the shades where possible. Do not make it completely dark, as this may be frightening for some children.
- Complementary therapies may be added, where appropriate, to enhance the experience—especially for meditation!—Aromatherapy, reflexology, or massage, are some suggestions worth exploring.

- Journaling or crafting is encouraged, especially following meditation and relaxation exercises. This allows children to explore their inner consciousness and the effects the practice has on their mind and body. It can also be enlightening for parents and teachers.
- Most of the techniques are adaptable for all ages. Use discretion and adapt accordingly.
- Most techniques are transferable – meaning they do not need to be practiced in an ideal or perfect place. Use discretion, yet be creative and teach kids how to use these techniques anywhere and time the need arises – for example, long lines at the movies or amusement park.
- Keep a box of tissues on hand, sinuses can be stimulated when practicing breathing techniques and tissues may be needed to help clear them out – be sure to tell the children this may happen and give them permission to help themselves to the tissue box as needed before commencing.

Posture Guide

Poor posture leads to an unhealthy muscular and skeletal system, and can negatively impact circulation, digestion, breathing and self-esteem. When practicing breathing and relaxation techniques you need access to your full breathing system – nose, mouth, throat, lungs, diaphragm, chest, back, and belly. If you were slouching in a chair, or curled in a ball on the sofa, do you think your body positions would allow access to all of those areas, giving you enough space to breath naturally and freely? No way!

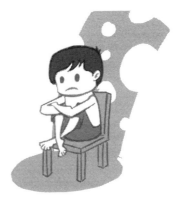

Poor Posture

Good posture allows access to our full breathing apparatus while practicing breathing techniques. With time, your general posture will naturally improve creating space in the body for better breathing on a daily basis, along with a host of additional health benefits. It is also very important to feel comfortable, supported, and relaxed while practicing breathing and relaxation techniques, and to eliminate physical strain, which only adds to or creates tension.

The following guide demonstrates postures recommended for seated, standing or supine practice, along with the recommended use of bolsters, blankets, and props to ensure comfort and support no matter how you choose to practice.

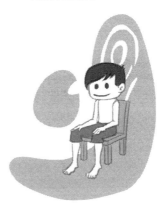

Good Posture

Seated on Floor:

CRISSCROSS:

- Sit on the floor or a yoga mat crisscross with one ankle in front of the other.
- Allow knees to fall out to the sides.
- Rest hands on the thighs and be sure the shoulders are relaxed – imagine both shoulder blades sliding down your back as the shoulders relax away from the ears.
- Gently press the sit bones in to the floor and feel the spine float to an erect position as you do so. This should feel very natural and not forced, the spine and body upright but not rigid.
- Keep the chin level with the floor.
- Scan the body and be sure you are not holding tension anywhere while maintaining this posture. Remain erect yet relaxed.

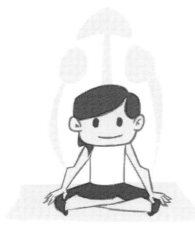

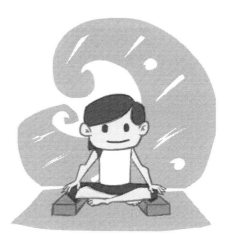

Crisscross   Supported Crisscross

Adjustments:

- Placing a folded up blanket, yoga block, cushion or pillow under the butt helps to support the spine, hips and knees in this position. It can also be more comfortable on your tush!
- Additional support can be added under the knees where needed – use blocks, bolsters, or folded blankets.

Tip: When sitting crisscross switch which leg is in front each time you sit. You will gravitate toward your dominant side, but by switching you help to maintain balance in the hips and strengthen your non-dominant side.

KNEES:

- Kneel on the floor or yoga mat, sitting on your heels, hands resting on the thighs.
- Be sure the shoulders are relaxed – imagine both shoulder blades sliding down your back as the shoulders relax away from the ears.
- Chin should be level and spine naturally erect. The spine and body upright, but not rigid.

Adjustment:

If this puts too much strain on the knees, do not sit on your heels. Place a yoga block or bolster between the calves and sit on it. You will still be kneeling, but your butt will be on the prop while the calves and feet frame the prop (see picture).

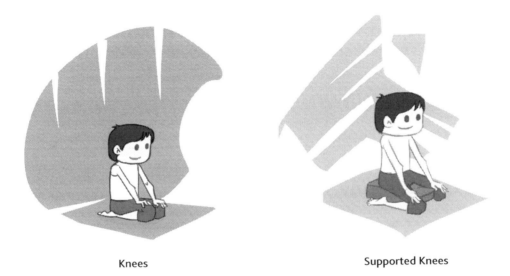

Knees   Supported Knees

*Tip: If you find you are slouching or are having trouble sitting up straight in any of the floor-seated postures, try sitting against a wall, or use a chair.

Seated Against Wall:

Find a clear wall space, without anything on it such as artwork or shelving.

- Place a folded blanket or bolster against the wall to sit on. Once seated, walk the butt back to make contact with the wall.
- Fold the legs into crisscross with one ankle in front of the other. If this is difficult or uncomfortable, sit with the legs extended straight out.
- Relax the back against the wall, allowing it to support the torso.
- Rest hands in lap and relax the shoulders - imagine both shoulder blades sliding down your back as the shoulders relax away from the ears.
- Gently press the sit bones in to the floor or bolster and feel the spine grow tall, this should feel very natural and not forced.
- Keep the chin level with the floor, remain relaxed and allow the wall to help support you.

Adjustment:

Place a pillow, bolster, or folded blanket between the lumbar spine and the wall where needed for extra support.

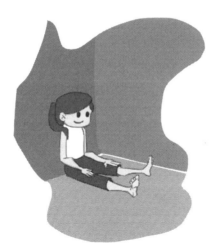

Against Wall

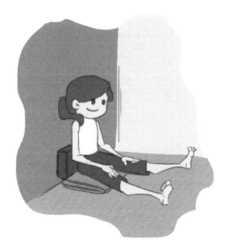

Supported Against Wall

Seated on Chair:

You will need a sturdy chair with a straight back for support.

- Sit on the chair with both feet planted firmly on the floor in front of it – you may need to scoot forward on the chair in order to reach the floor comfortably with both feet.
- Rest hands on the thighs and be sure the shoulders are relaxed – imagine both shoulder blades sliding down your back as the shoulders relax away from the ears.
- Gently press the sit bones in to the chair and feel the spine float to an erect position as you do so, this should feel very natural and not forced.
- Keep the chin level with the floor.
- Scan the body and be sure you are not holding tension anywhere while maintaining this posture.
- Remain erect yet relaxed, the spine and body upright, but not rigid.

Adjustment:

If the lumbar support or back of chair does not support your back – it may not reach when both feet are on the floor – place a pillow, bolster or blanket between the back of chair and the torso for additional support.

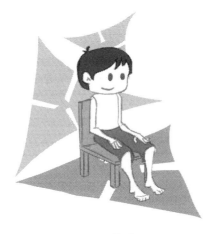

Chair

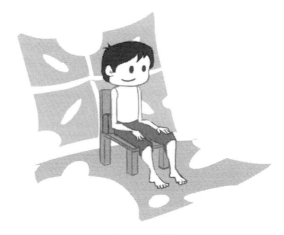

Supported Chair

Standing:

When practicing breathing or relaxation techniques standing, stand solid, strong and still, like a mountain. Build your mountain like this:

- Begin standing with feet hip-width distance apart.
- Press both feet evenly in to the floor and feel the sternum slightly pull up as the spine floats to a naturally erect position.
- Rest the arms alongside the torso and be sure the shoulders are relaxed – imagine both shoulder blades sliding down your back as the shoulders relax away from the ears.
- Palms face forward with the fingers spread like stars.
- Allow the chin to be level with the floor.
- Scan the body and be sure you are not holding tension anywhere while maintaining this posture. Remain upright yet relaxed, not rigid… just like a mountain!

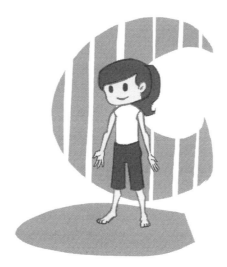

Mountain

Supine:

The supine posture and adjustments described below are for practice while lying on a yoga mat or the floor; they can be adapted for use on a bed or sofa where necessary.

- Begin lying on the floor.
- Hug the knees into the chest and feel the spine flatten along the floor.
- Release legs, one at a time, stretching them out along the floor.
- Allow the feet to fall open, relaxed.
- Tuck the shoulder blades under one at a time – this opens the chest and front side of torso — then relax the shoulders and upper body on the floor.
- Allow the arms to rest on the floor alongside the torso.
- Hands rest with the palms facing up, or they can fold in and rest palms down on the belly.
- Let go of any muscle engagement and allow the floor to fully support the body.

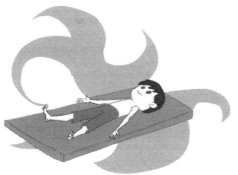

Supine

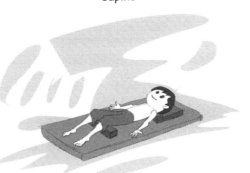

Supported Supine

Adjustments:

- Support and protect the lower back by placing a pillow, rolled up blanket or bolster just below the knees, OR, bend the knees so they point toward the ceiling and place the feet flat on the floor, a few inches from the hips and hip-width distance apart. Knees can fall in, resting against one another, or remain separated.
- Support the head and neck by using a pillow or folded up blanket under the head.

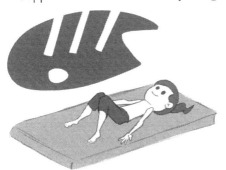

Knees Bent, Lean In

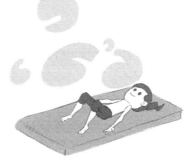

Knees Bent, Open

Breath Play

Introduction: *Breath Play*

Explore the breath and how it works with *Breath Play*, a series of fun activities and games for kids of all ages. Actively engaging, *Breath Play* allows kids to see and feel their breath, cultivating an awareness of how it works in their own bodies. Through play they discover that altering or controlling the breath can change and effect the way they feel.

Explode like a firework, sing like an opera singer, or roar like a lion – the activities and games in *Breath Play* capture the imagination while harnessing excess energy, releasing tension, and relieving physical and/or mental stress. Centering and calming, they promote relaxation by encouraging full, deep breaths that calm the nervous system.

Perfect for the mid-afternoon slump period, some exercises are energizing and stretch and flex the physical body. Additional benefits include the development of patience, coordination, focus, concentration, self-esteem, confidence, independence, self-regulation, and, teamwork and cooperation.

Go ahead, breathe, play, laugh and learn. Most importantly, have FUN!

Guidelines

Once playtime is over, encourage an open discussion allowing the children to explore and acknowledge any differences noticed in the way they breathed and how they felt in their minds and bodies after playing the games.

Breath Play exercises are especially useful to demonstrate how the breath works and how to control it before moving on to teaching *Breathing Techniques*.

Caution

Young kids can get a little overzealous when first learning any type of breathing technique. Start slow when introducing breathing activities, and incrementally build the time practiced or number of reps as their skills develop. Encourage smooth, even, controlled breaths that are never forced.

Hoberman Sphere

What is a Hoberman Sphere?

A Hoberman Sphere is a plastic, dome shaped toy with a hinge-like joint action that allows it to fold down to a small compact ball and expand out to a large sphere shape.

How does it help me?

A Hoberman Sphere can be used as a visual tool to help you connect to your breath by observing it. Your lungs are very similar to a Hoberman Sphere given they expand when you inhale and contract when you exhale. Linking the simple expansion and contraction of the Hoberman Sphere to your own inhales and exhales serves as a visual aid to observe your breath, enabling you to work toward slowing and deepening the breath as well as learning how to "even out" the breath – inhaling and exhaling smoothly and for an equal count.

How do I do it?

- Begin in a comfortable seated position, sitting up tall but relaxed.
- As you breathe in, slowly expand the Hoberman Sphere for the duration of your inhale. Once your inhale is complete, stop expanding the Hoberman Sphere.
- Notice the natural pause between your inhale and exhale.
- As you begin to exhale, collapse the Hoberman Sphere until your exhale is complete. Stop and notice the natural pause before your inhale begins. Repeat.
- Notice how far you expand the sphere as you inhale. Does the sphere move all of the way back to the same starting point when you complete your exhale? If not, work toward making the movement of the Hoberman Sphere—and your inhale and exhale—even.

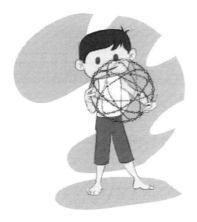
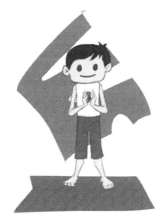

Inhale – Expand   Exhale – Contract

No Hoberman Sphere? No problem!

Use your hands if you do not have access to a Hoberman Sphere! Begin with the palms pressed together in front of your torso. Breathe in, slowly moving the palms away from one another, stopping when you complete your inhale. Notice the natural pause between your inhale and exhale. As you exhale, slowly move the palms back to meet each other. Was your inhale as long as your exhale? Did your hands meet back together at the end of your exhale? Work toward making this happen.

*Tip: Once you have mastered evening out your inhales and exhales, and you feel very comfortable with this type of breathing (i.e. it feels natural and not forced), challenge yourself by learning to extend your exhale, that is make your exhale last a little longer than your inhale. Build very slowly, incrementally making your exhale longer and longer, but never make the exhale last more than two times the inhale. (Learn more about "Lengthening the Exhale" in *Breathing Techniques*).

Pinwheel Breathing

What is Pinwheel Breathing?

We all have the power and strength of the wind within us and prove it when we play with pinwheels! Blowing hard we make them spin wild and fast, but can we make them spin slowly and steadily for a long time? ... Of course we can!

How does it help me?

Pinwheels are a FUN way to explore the breath and how we can control it in ways that benefit our mind and our body. Playing with pinwheels we teach ourselves to extend the out breath (exhale) and discover how this can lead to feelings of relaxation.

How do I do it?

You will need a pinwheel – you can buy these at a dollar store, or if you are feeling creative you can make one (a quick visit to craft websites should turn up a pinwheel how-to craft).

- Begin in a comfortable seated position.
- Take a deep breath in through the nose and bring pinwheel a few inches from your mouth.
- Gently exhale, blowing the pinwheel so it moves.
- How fast did your pinwheel move? How long did it spin for?
- Take another breath in and blow on your pinwheel again. Can you make your exhale last for a long time so your pinwheel spins even longer than last time?
- Play around with it and make your pinwheel spin at different speeds?

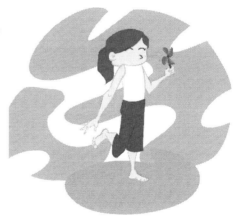

Pinwheel Breathing

- Notice how your body feels when you make the pinwheel spin for a long time versus when you make it spin fast.
- Notice which parts of your body are active when you change the way you breathe.
- Which breath makes you feel calm and relaxed?

Bubbles

What are Bubbles?

Bubbles are a fun way to explore the breath and how it can help us to relax and feel good.

How does it help me?

Providing a great visual, Bubbles are an excellent way to learn about your breath by physically seeing what happens when you breathe differently. As you play, you will learn what type of breathing makes you feel better and more relaxed. And who doesn't want to have some fun while they learn?

What do I need?

- Bubble wand
- Liquid soap

*Tip: For extra fun you can try colored bubbles (Crayola) or bubbles that don't pop easily (Gymboree).

How do I do it?

- Swirl your bubble wand in liquid soap and then hold it a few inches from your lips.
- Gently blow through pursed lips as you watch your bubble grow.
- Try blowing a sharp burst of air and see if you can make a bubble this way.
- What works best? Blowing a long gentle, steady stream of air, or a short powerful burst?
- Notice how these two different breaths make you feel? Notice which parts of your body engage or relax with each breath?

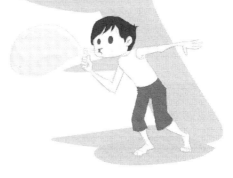

Bubbles

- Which is easier?
- Which breath makes the biggest bubbles?
- HAVE FUN! Make as many big, beautiful bubbles as you can.
- FEEL GOOD! Notice how slowly blowing bubbles makes you feel super-relaxed.

*Tip: Bubbles can leave a sticky residue on the floor or leave a slippery mess. Be sure to blow bubbles in an area that won't get messed up and is safe, like outside with adult supervision.

Bubbles in Milk

What is Bubbles in Milk?

Bubbles in Milk is a FUN way to learn about the breath. Kids of all ages love this – even big kids (especially those who, like me, were told not to do this as a child!).

How does it help me?

Learning to breathe deeply and with control is very important. Blowing Bubbles in Milk creates a strong visual, allowing you to actually see when long, controlled exhales are at work and when they are not. An activity that is fun and educational – what more could you ask for?

What do I need?

- Plastic Cup
- Straw
- Milk (almond milk bubbles up very well)

How do I do it?

- Fill the plastic cup a little less than halfway with milk.
- Place the straw in the cup.
- Take a full breath in through your nose and, once you have completed your inhale, place the straw in your mouth, gently pursing the lips around it.
- Slowly exhale through the straw with control and watch the bubbles form.
- The best way to make lots of bubbles is to blow into the straw very slowly for as long of possible.
- Play around with it, blow hard and see the difference in the type of bubbles this creates. Notice how quickly the bubbles dissipate. Do you notice any difference between those created with a long, slow exhale compared with those made with short, sharp bursts of air?
- Have FUN!

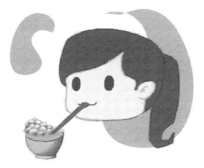

Bubbles in Milk

Singing Breath

What is Singing Breath and how does it help me?

Singing Breath is a fun way to make some noise and release tension. It also helps bring awareness to your breath, teaching you to breath fully and deeply which promotes relaxation.

How do I do it?

As an example we will use the vowel sounds of the alphabet (A-E-I-O-U) to describe this exercise, but you can use any sounds at all! Singing your name or the name of a friend, or even something as simple as *"do, re, mi"*…. The only rules are to have fun, and to use the entire out breath (or exhale) to make your sound.

- Take a big breath in, filling up your lungs. Sweep your arms up overhead as you breathe in, this allows more space for the ribs to expand, resulting in a fuller "in breath" or inhale.

- Open your mouth and exhale by singing the letter "A" until all of the air is out of your body. Like this, "Aaaaaaaaaaaaaaaaaaaaaaaaaaaaaaaaaaaaaaaaa…". The sound should stop once you have emptied all of the air from your lungs. Float the arms back down by your sides as you sing the sound.

- Take another deep breath in, sweeping the arms up overhead, and repeat with the next vowel, "Eeeeeeeeeeeeeeeeeeeeeee…". And so on.

*Tip: Don't be afraid to make noise or laugh, making noise and laughing are great ways to release tension from the body. Have fun with this.

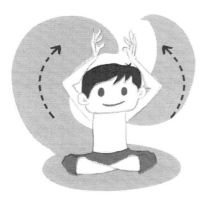

INHALE

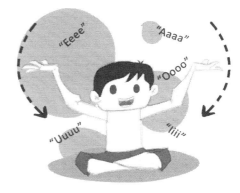

EXHALE

Feel the Vibration

What is Feel the Vibration?

Feel the Vibration is a fun technique that teaches us how we use our breath and body in different ways to make certain sounds.

How does it help me?

Developing an awareness of the breath and our ability to control it is an important aspect of the mind-body connection. This exercise demonstrates that just as we can make sounds at will, we have the ability to bring a sense of relaxation and calm to our bodies and minds by using our breath.

How do I do it?

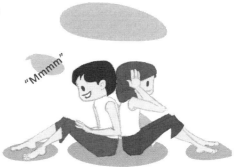

- Begin in a comfortable seated position, spine naturally erect. Feet flat on the floor, shoulders and arms relaxed, hands resting in the lap.
- Begin humming the "Mmmm" sound. Notice where you feel it most (for this sound, it will most likely be the lips and mouth).
- Continue making the sound and scan the body for other areas the sound is effecting – it may be less obvious than the lips in the case of "Mmmm", it may be the throat or even further down in the abdominal area. For example, you may also feel the belly pulling in as you make the "Mmmm" sound.

Feel the Vibration Partner Exercise

- Play around with different sounds and really examine each one, first for where you feel it in the body the most, followed by the more subtle areas.
- Where does the sound originate? Where does it end? What muscles engage? Do any relax? How does each sound differ from the others? Are some similar in regards to their effect on the body?
- HAVE FUN!

*Tip: Try this sitting back to back with a friend or partner. Notice how each sound feels coming from a different person. Play a game – place both fingers in your ears and see if you can guess which sound your partner is making based on the vibration and movement you feel coming from their body. Switch and take turns.

SOME SOUNDS TO TRY:

LONG: "Aahh", "Vvvv", "Oohh", "Aayy", "Eeee", "Iiii", "Oooo", "Yoou", "Ssss", "Zzzz", "Sshh", "Hmmm", "Laaa"…

SHORT: "Hah", "Uh", "Ugh", "The", "Ba", "Pa", "La", "Do", "Doh", "Ga", "Car"…

Bumblebee Breath

What is Bumblebee Breath?

Bumblebee Breath is a fun breathing technique where you make the sound of a bumblebee. Tickling your mouth and lips, Bumblebee Breath fills your whole body with the vibration and energy of your own breath.

How does it help me?

Bumblebee Breath helps shift our attention inwardly by shutting off outside distractions and focusing on the vibration of our own breath. A soothing practice, it results in feelings of relaxation and calm. Bumblebee Breath is also empowering, reminding us of the power and energy we already have inside of us.

How do I do it?

- Begin in a comfortable seated position, either on the floor or in a chair. Sit up nice and tall, but relaxed.

- Place your thumbs in your ears, blocking any outside sounds; gently wrap the remaining four fingers over closed eyes, this will help you really focus on what is happening inside of you.

- Take a big breath in, filling up with air until the belly expands. Exhale through the nose keeping your lips closed, making a humming sound for the duration of your exhale.

- Keeping your eyes closed, return to normal breathing and gently rest your hands in your lap. Observe the sensations the sound has created in your body.

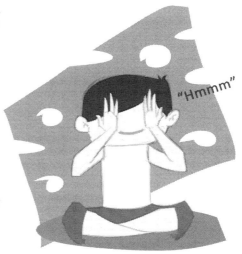

"Hmmm"

Bumblebee Breath

- Repeat for several rounds, gradually building to 5-10 rounds per sitting.

- If you feel dizzy or light-headed while practicing Bumblebee Breath (or any breathing exercise), take a break and resume normal breathing.

Discussion: What did you feel when you practiced Bumblebee Breath? Did you feel the buzzing sensation or vibration anywhere else, or only your lips? How about your tongue? What happened when the breath and sound finished? Could you still feel the vibration? How did it make you feel after? Did your mind or thoughts wander while you were practicing Bumblebee Breath?

Feather Breath

What is Feather Breath?

Feather Breath utilizes fun games and colorful feathers to learn more about how we breathe and how we can change our breath to make us feel more relaxed or more energized.

What do I need to play?

- Feathers
- Straws

How do I do it?

Seeing the Breath:

- Rest a single feather in the open palm of your hand, holding it just below the chin.
- Breathe normally.
- Watch the feather closely and notice how it moves. You are observing your inhale and exhale as the feather moves. Can you tell which is your inhale and which is your exhale based on the movement of the feather?

Exhaling:

Now that you know what your breath looks like and that it can move the feather even when you are breathing normally, let's explore how exhaling can feel different, not only for the feather, but for you!

- Hold the feather upright, placing the stem between your thumb and index finger.
- Notice how the feather has soft, light plumes, while other parts of the feather are stiff.
- Use your breath to move only the soft parts of the feather.
- Now use the breath to move the stiffer parts.
- What do you notice about the way you must exhale to move the soft parts of the feather? And the stiff? How does each exhale make you feel?
- Play around some more with this and notice which parts of your body move when making the different breaths. Where does the breath originate? Which body parts relax or contract?
- Which exhale makes you feel good?

Feather Storm:

Not unlike a great pile of leaves following a fall leaf storm, feather storms are fun to play in with your friends. You will need two or more people, one straw for each person, and a small (or large) pile of feathers to place on the floor between you.

- Lie on your bellies on the floor with the feathers scattered in the middle.
- Blow through the straws, aiming at the feathers to make them rise up and swirl around.
- Can you keep the storm blowing? Can you work together to make sure none of the feathers fly outside of the circle?
- Does one type of exhale help you play this game better? If so, which one?

Feather Float:

To play Feather Float you will need a straw and a feather.

- Toss the feather high up into the air and blow through the straw to keep the feather off the ground.
- If playing in a group, the person who keeps the feather from hitting the ground longest is the winner.
- If playing individually, time yourself and keep trying to beat your own time by keeping the feather in the air as long as you can.
- What kind of exhale helps you play this game better?

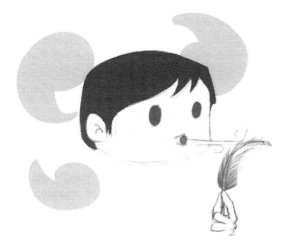

Feather Breath

Water Wheel

What is Water Wheel?

Water Wheel is an active breathing exercise that engages the physical body in a pump-like action.

How does it help me?

Similar to the action the diaphragm makes when breathing, the physical movement the body makes practicing Water Wheel encourages full diaphragmatic breathing. Water Wheel actively engages the abdominals, so you get a little bit of a core work out too – a strong core supports your lower back and helps maintain good posture, which allows you to breath better. The physical pumping action of the legs in this exercise encourages you to take deeper and fuller breaths.

How do I do it?

- Begin lying on your back.
- Hug your knees in to your chest and press your lower back in to the floor. Keep both hips in contact with the floor the entire time you practice Water Wheel.
- Slide your hands to the tops of the knees, and as you inhale drop your feet toward the floor, just below the hips.
- Exhale and hug the knees back in to the chest, squeezing all of the air out of your lungs as you hug the knees in.
- Inhale and slowly lower the feet back to the floor.
- Exhale and draw knees back in toward the chest.
- Repeat for several rounds, rhythmic and smooth movements like a water wheel pumping in synch with your breath.

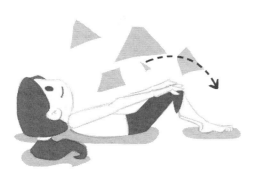

INHALE

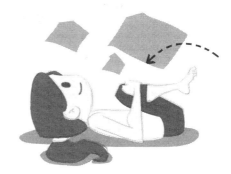

EXHALE

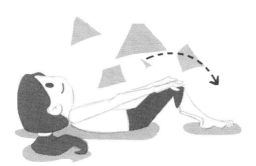

INHALE

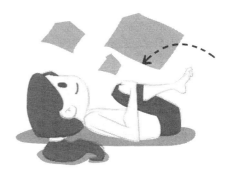

EXHALE

Balloon Breath

What is Balloon Breath?

Balloon Breath is a breathing technique that slows the breath down while encouraging full and deep inhales and exhales to calm the mind and body.

How does it help me?

Balloon Breath is centering and calming. It is great to use as a quick exercise to center and calm oneself during activities or to refocus before or during class. Linking physical movement to the breath encourages mind-body connection, a form of meditation or present moment awareness resulting in relaxation and a deep sense of calm. The physical movement of raising the arms up overhead in this exercise allows more space in the torso to accommodate fuller and deeper breaths.

How do I do it?

- Begin sitting comfortably, either on a chair or on the floor with the hands resting on the thighs, the shoulders, arms, and face should be relaxed.
- OR, begin standing, feet hip width distance apart, arms resting by the torso, shoulders and face relaxed.
- Begin to breathe in and out through the nose.
- Inhale, sweeping your arms up overhead and imagine you are filling up a giant balloon.
- Exhale, slowly lowering your arms to rest in your lap or by your side.
- Repeat for several rounds.
- Get CREATIVE: Imagine the color of your balloon as you inflate it. Does thinking of a certain color make you feel more relaxed?
- Get CREATIVE: Imagine releasing your balloon off into the sky as you exhale. Where does your balloon go?

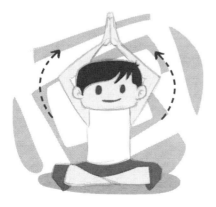

INHALE

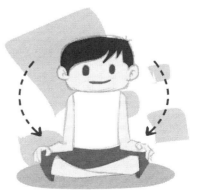

EXHALE

People Powered Plane

What is People Powered Plane?

Exploring our breath is fun, especially when we do it with our friends. People Powered Plane is a game to be played with a small group of friends that reaps the many benefits of deep breathing and linking movement to breath.

How does it help me?

Working together is teamwork, and flying our plane together while breathing in unison teaches us that TOGETHER we can do anything! The physical movements made in People Powered Plane teach co-ordination skills while creating space in the torso to allow deeper breathing to occur.

How do I do it?

- Sit on the knees, one person behind the other in a row, all facing the same direction.
- Inhale together - flapping your arms in a gentle and slow up and down motion as you slowly rise to stand on knees. At top of your inhale you should be standing on your knees with your arms stretched up overhead.
- Exhale together - flapping your arms in a gentle and slow up and down motion as you slowly lower to sit back on your heels. At the end of your exhale, you should be kneeling, sitting on your heels, with the arms resting by your side.
- That is one round. Repeat up to 5 full rounds of in breaths and out breaths.

*Tip: In the beginning it may be difficult to time your own inhales and exhales with those of your friends. This is okay, we all breathe differently – as long as you are doing your best and following your own breath without forcing it or straining it. Eventually, you will fall into a rhythm with your friends where you are all breathing – and flying – at a similar pace.

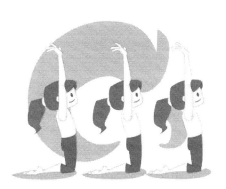

INHALE

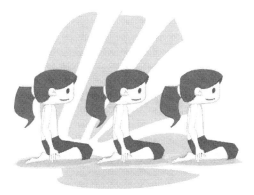

EXHALE

Elephant Shower

What is Elephant Shower and how does it help me?

Elephant Shower is an active breathing posture that has a stretching component to stretch and energize your body, and a releasing component that encourages relaxation and a sense of letting go. The releasing part of Elephant Shower is actually a type of physical inversion, meaning your head is lower than your heart, inversions are known to be rejuvenating. Elephant shower is great to use when you feel fidgety and have a lot of excess energy – it is a positive way to release some of that energy, center yourself, stretch, relax, and feel good.

How do I do it?

- Begin standing with your feet slightly wider than hip width distance apart.
- Link your hands together to make a trunk with your arms.
- Fold at your hips and allow your head and arms to hang heavy.
- Pretend you have a huge waterhole at your feet and drink some water up through your trunk – make slurping sounds as you slurp water into your trunk!
- When you have had enough to drink, take a BIG breath in as you take one final slurp through your trunk.
- As you exhale, stand up tall, lifting your trunk high up in the air over your head – spraying the water like a shower.
- Take a big breath in, stretching your trunk high over your head.
- As you breathe out, lower your trunk, folding your body over your legs, allowing your arms and head hang heavy.
- Repeat for 3 rounds.
- Get CREATIVE: Imagine your elephant is showering in something other than water. Your favorite color, happiness, glitter, or giggles! You can shower yourself with anything you like.
- Have FUN: Shower your friends with happiness, glitter and giggles too.

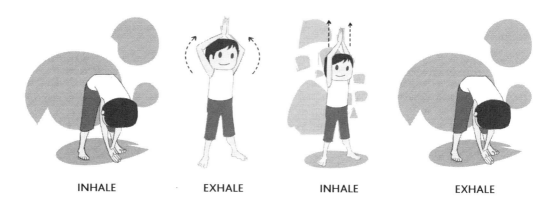

INHALE   EXHALE   INHALE   EXHALE

Air Soccer/Ball Pass

What is Air Soccer/Ball Pass?

Air Soccer and Ball Pass are fun games that can be played with friends that teach us how our breath can work in different ways to benefit our health and how we feel.

What do I need?

- Straws (thick smoothie straws or regular drinking straws)
- Pom-poms OR ping pong balls OR balled up tissue paper
- Shoe boxes OR small-medium sized boxes (empty, no lids)

How do I play?

One Player:

- Lay a shoebox on its side with the open part facing in. Set it at one end of yoga mat or room, this is your "goal".
- Lie on your belly at the other end of the yoga mat, or room. Have a straw and pom-pom (or ball or balled up paper) with you.
- Gently blow into the straw to move your pom-pom down the mat and into the "goal". Play against yourself and see if you can get the ball into the goal with the least amount of breaths. Challenge yourself by placing the goal further away from your starting point each time.

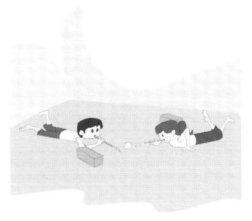

Air Soccer

Two or More Players:

- Pass the pom-pom back and forth between players.
- Set up "goals" at each end of floor area and allocate one goal to each team. Work together with your teammates to score goals and to stop the opposing team from scoring goals. The team with the most goals after a certain time period will be declared the winning team. (To avoid too much chaos, allocate one area of the playing field per player, including a goalie for each team. If there are only two players, they may cover full area.)

*Tip: The aim is to have control over the direction your pom-pom rolls – short bursts of breath will send it flying, but you won't have control. Deep inhales with long controlled exhales will help you direct your ball toward the goals and away from the opposition team! Notice how breathing this way makes you feel.

Golf

What is Golf and how does it help me?

A variation of the breath game Air Soccer, Golf is a fun way to learn about the breath and train the body to breathe fully and deeply. Focusing on lengthening the out-breath (or exhale) – something you will need to score a hole in one! – Golf benefits its players by slowing the breath down, calming the nervous system, and cultivating awareness of the breath and how it can consciously be changed to benefit the body (and your Golf score!).

What will I need?

- A clear floor space, or several yoga mats lined up side by side to create one large surface area.
- Beanbags or cones to use as markers.
- Straws (bendy ones are easier for kids to maneuver at floor-level).
- Pompoms or ping-pong balls (balled up tissue can be used if you don't have pompoms or ping-pong balls).

How do I do it?

- Set markers in zigzag pattern on floor area.
- Player one moves their ball or pom-pom toward the first marker by blowing air through their straw.
- Once player one passes the first marker, player two can begin. (Players move toward each marker once the player in front of them has passed it).
- The object is for each player to count how many times they blow the ball between markers, and to work toward getting the ball from one marker to the next using one breath – a hole in one!
- Players play against themselves, playing the course several times working toward improving their score.

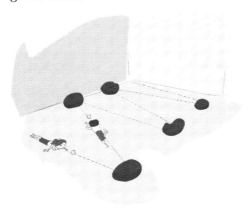

Golf

Snorkel Breath

What is Snorkel Breath and how does it help me?

Similar to a pipe or straw, a snorkel enables a swimmer to keep his or her face submerged in the water, observing fish, coral or sea-life, and to breathe at the same time. Snorkel Breath is a technique that uses a straw to emphasize a full exhale, triggering a naturally occurring deeper inhale.

How do I do it?

- Use a regular drinking straw – not a supersize smoothie straw – the bendy straws are fun to use as they can be bent into the shape of a "snorkel".
- Take a full breath in through your nose and, once you have completed your inhale, place the straw in your mouth, gently pursing the lips around it.
- Slowly exhale through the straw.
- Once your exhale is complete, remove the straw and breathe normally for a couple of cycles before repeating.
- Practice Snorkel Breath for a few rounds, building on the number of cycles you complete each time you practice.

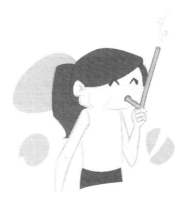

Snorkel Breath

Creative Games:

Scatter images of sea creatures (foam shapes, flash cards, plastic figurines). Take a breath in, put your snorkel on (straw in your mouth) and breath out. As you breath out, pick a random sea creature. Remove your "snorkel" and create a shape with your body based on the sea creature you "discovered on your snorkel trip".

Horse Breath

What is Horse Breath?

Horse Breath is a breathing technique also known as pursed lip breathing. While it is a lot of fun to do, this exercise is more than mere horseplay and boasts plenty of health benefits.

How does it help me?

Horse Breath is an excellent exercise to regulate your breathing if you find yourself short of breath. Engagement of the abdominal muscles during the exhale causes a deeper exhale to occur, this will automatically be followed by a deeper inhale – regulating and slowing the breath down. Horse Breath also relaxes the mouth and jaw area, places we commonly carry tension without being aware of it!

How do I do it?

- Begin in a comfortable seated position.
- Take a normal inhale through the nose (does not need to be a deep inhale).
- Keep the lips relaxed and in a rested position (closed but not closed tightly), and exhale through the mouth. The lips should vibrate and flop around as the air passes through them.
- Inhale through the nose and repeat for a few rounds, building to 3-5 rounds per session.
- Observe the rest of your body when you breathe this way. Do you feel your abdominals engage as you exhale? Do you notice that you naturally breathe a little deeper after practicing Horse Breath for a few rounds? How does it make you feel?

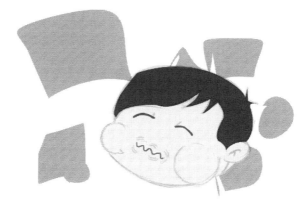

Horse Breath

Lion's Breath

What is Lion's Breath and how does it help me?

Lion's Breath is a fantastic exercise to release tension and stress. It stretches the mouth, jaw, tongue, eyes and hands – all common areas where tension can be found. Practicing Lion's Breath is also a lot of fun.

How do I do it?

- Begin by kneeling on the floor, sitting upright, spine naturally erect. If sitting on the knees is too uncomfortable for your joints, sitting in a chair is fine – be sure to be sitting nice and straight with both feet planted on the floor. Hands should be relaxed, resting comfortably on the lap.
- Inhale deeply through your nose.
- Open your mouth wide, stick your tongue out and exhale strongly while making a "Haaaa" sound.
- Turn eyes to look up toward the ceiling and stretch hands and fingers to frame either side of your face like a lion's bushy mane.
- Repeat 2-3 times.
- Notice how you feel after practicing Lion's Breath.

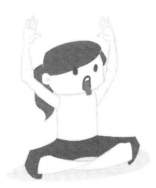

Lion's Breath

Funny Bunny Breath

What is Funny Bunny Breath?

Funny Bunny Breath is an energizing breath exercise.

How does it help me?

Funny Bunny Breath serves as a quick pick me up when you feel a little sluggish. The quick intake of oxygen revives the mind and body, BUT take care not to over do it. NEVER complete more than 3-5 rounds of Funny Bunny Breath at one time, and SLOWLY build to this, beginning with just one round.

How do I do it?

- Begin sitting on the knees, if kneeling is uncomfortable or difficult sit crisscross on the floor or upright in a chair.
- Rest your hands on your thighs.
- Exhale fully through the mouth making an "Aahh" sound until all the air is out.
- Close your mouth, wrinkle your nose like a bunny sniffing around a carrot and take three quick inhalations through the nose.
- Open the mouth and exhale fully with an, "Aahh" sound.
- As you gain experience and become comfortable with this breathing technique, build to 3-5 rounds of Funny Bunny Breath per session as needed. Remember to *slowly* build to a higher number of rounds when practicing any breathing technique.

Firework Breath

What is Firework Breath?

Firework Breath is a fun, active breathing exercise that is great for shaking off excess energy or silliness.

How does it help me?

Sometimes we have a lot of excess energy buzzing around inside of us, making it really hard to focus or concentrate on important things, like schoolwork. Firework Breath uses the body and the breath to harness and release some of that energy, making it easy for you to sit, focus, do great work and learn.

How do I do it?

- Bending the knees, lower into a squat position.
- Draw your hands to heart center with the palms pressed together. This is the tip of your firework launcher.
- Take a deep breath in through the nose, filling up your lungs.
- Launch your firework! Keep your palms pressed into each other as you shoot your arms straight up like a missile and jump to a standing position, then spread the arms and legs out wide, like an exploding Firework. Breathe out loudly through an open mouth as your firework explodes, "Paah…!".
- Imagine what color and type of firework you are. Imagine how bright and dynamic you are.

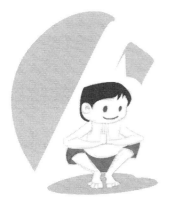

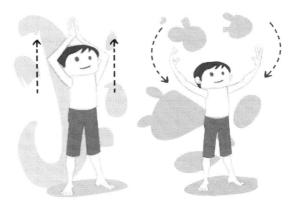

INHALE   EXHALE

Locomotive

What is Locomotive?

Locomotive is a fun, active breathing exercise that also gently stretches and flexes the spine. Linking movement to the breath and making the sounds of a train, also makes Locomotive a present moment awareness exercise.

How does it help me?

Gently flexing and stretching the spine allows for better movement and mobility, and better posture. Having good posture is healthy for our skeletal and muscular systems and creates space in our torso so we can breathe fully and deeply. Practicing Locomotive also has meditative benefits, matching the movement to the breath connects the mind and the body, while the "chhh" sound made while exhaling is great for releasing tension from the body.

How do I do it?

- Begin in a comfortable seated position, either sitting on the knees or crisscross on the floor, or seated on a chair.
- Rest hands, palms facing down, on thighs or knees.
- As you inhale through your nose, push your chest and belly forward as your butt and shoulders curl back, making a "c" shape with your spine.
- Exhale through your lips, making a "chhh" sound, as you pull your belly-button in toward your spine, tuck your tailbone and chin, and curl your spine into a "c" shape in the opposite direction.
- Repeat for several rounds.
- Play around with making your train travel at different speeds and notice how it makes you feel.

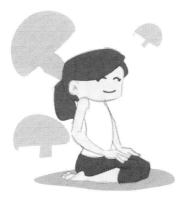

INHALE

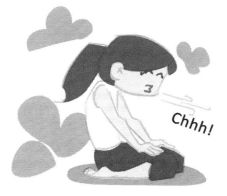

Chhh!

EXHALE

Thunderstorm

What is Thunderstorm and how does it help me?

Thunderstorm is a fun way to work all of the tension out of your body, preparing you for relaxation. It is also a great way to harness and release any extra energy you may have, preparing you to settle in and focus on something important such as a class or test.

How do I do it?

- Begin sitting on knees and lightly tap on legs, torso, shoulders and head with fingertips. The rain is beginning to lightly fall.
- Increase the tapping as the rain becomes harder.
- Lightly pat the floor with the palms as the rain becomes even harder. (Alternating the palms will create the sound of rain.)
- Come onto the thighs, patting the thighs creating the sound of even stronger rainfall.
- Pound the palms onto the floor – making thunder. (Pounding both palms at same time will simulate thunder.)
- Sit up and skim the palms together in an up and down motion to make lightening.
- Switch between Rain – palms alternating on tops of the thighs or the floor, Thunder – palms pounding the floor, and Lightening – palms skimming up and down.
- Begin to slow the rain back down to a sprinkle. Rain drops getting lighter and lighter with each moment.
- Stretch out on the floor like a big, giant puddle left over from the storm and rest for up to five minutes.

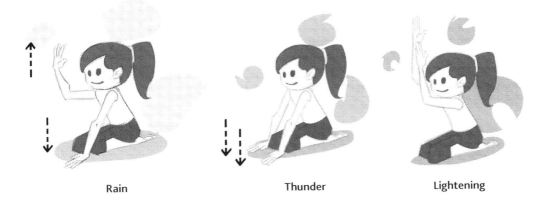

Rain   Thunder   Lightening

*Variations: Spaghetti Boil and Milk Shake - try these additional, fun variations of this relaxation technique for kids!

Milk Shake

What is Milk Shake and how does it help me?

Milk Shake is a fun way to shake any tension out of your body, preparing you for relaxation. It is also a great way to harness and release any extra energy, anxiety or silliness you may feel, preparing you to settle in and focus on something important such as a class or test.

How do I do it?

- First, imagine what ingredients you would like in your milkshake. You can put anything you like in it – for example, banana, yogurt and milk.
- Imagine the top of the blender is the top of your head, reach up and pour the milk inside your blender.
- Now add the yogurt.
- Stretch both hands overhead and lean to the right making a banana shape. Come back to center and stretch up tall before leaning to the left like a banana, when you come back to center, place the banana inside your blender.
- Gently pat the top of your head to be sure the lid is on.
- Turn the blender on and shake your milkshake! Shake your legs, shake your arms, wiggle your shoulders, and run on the spot. Shake-shake-shake your ingredients as fast as you can.
- Begin to slow your blender down, your movements becoming slower and slower.
- Lower your yummy, fluid milkshake onto the floor like a puddle. A giant puddle of banana milk shake – YUM!
- Stretch your body reaching your arms up overhead and point your toes – making a long straw out of your body to drink the milk shake with.

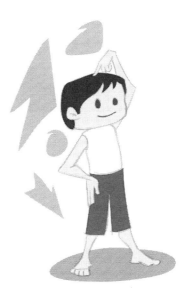

Put Ingredients in Blender

- Relax the entire body, resting your hands on your belly, full and happy after enjoying your yummy milk shake.
- Rest here for up to five minutes.

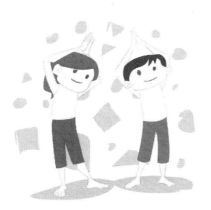

Banana Bend

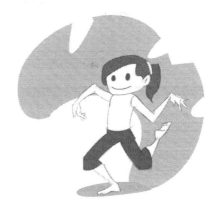

Milkshake

*Variations: Spaghetti Boil and Thunderstorm – try these additional, fun variations of this relaxation technique for kids!

Spaghetti Boil

What is Spaghetti Boil and how does it help me?

Spaghetti Boil is a fun way to shake all of the tension out of your body, preparing you for relaxation. It is also a positive way to harness and release any extra energy, anxieties, or silliness you may have, preparing you to settle in and focus on something important such as a class or test.

How do I do it?

- Begin standing up tall, arms relaxed by your side. Now stiffen yourself from fingertips to toes, like a hard, uncooked spaghetti noodle.
- Maintaining stiffness, slowly begin to walk in circle – arms and legs straight like a robot – your spaghetti noodle is still hard!
- Imagine the water in the pot getting warmer as it begins to boil. As the water gets warmer your spaghetti noodle gets softer.
- As the water builds to a boil, move a little faster in the circle.
- Once the water is boiling, your noodle should be soft and floppy and swirling around the pot, moving faster and faster. Your body loose and relaxed.
- Imagine the pot has been turned off and the boiling slows to a simmer. Slow the body down but stay floppy like a cooked noodle.
- Slowly lower your cooked noodle on to the floor and lie there all floppy.
- Rest for up to five minutes, allowing your noodle to cool down.

*Tip: Teachers can perform a cooked noodle test! Shake each child's limbs to test how floppy and well cooked their noodle is.

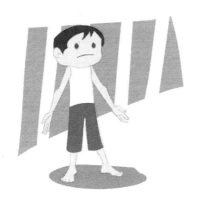
Uncooked Noodle

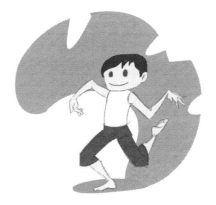
Cooked Noodle

*Variations: Milks Shake and Thunderstorm - try these additional, fun variations of this relaxation technique for kids!

Paint a Rainbow on the Sky*

*(Created by Allison Morgan, MA, OTR, RYT – *Zensational Kids, LLC*)

What is Paint a Rainbow on the Sky?

Paint a Rainbow on the Sky is an imagination based group activity to play with your friends that incorporates creative visualization, breathing, self-massage and teamwork.

How does it help me?

You and your friends will have fun, making a beautiful rainbow together and you will *all* feel nice and relaxed after.

How do I do it?

- Begin sitting in a small circle. Sit comfortably, either on the knees or in crisscross.
- Cup your hands in front of you to make a small bowl. Imagine – inside your mind, do not say it out loud! – the bowl of your hands being filled with any color paint you like. Be creative – it does not have to be a color traditionally found in a rainbow; it can be any color you like and can even have sparkles in it!
- Once you can picture the paint in your cupped hands, gently rub the palms of your hands together to mix the paint.

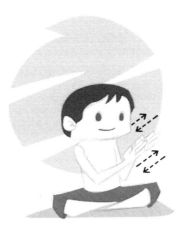

INHALE

- Now spread the paint by rubbing the paint up your arms, across your chest and shoulders, on your neck, face and head. Massage it into your hair and reach around to rub some on the back of your neck, rub it on your back and sides and on your belly. Rub it down your legs all of the way to your feet.
- Rub the palms together again to mix more paint in your special color, and as you do, take a deep breath in.
- As you breathe out, spread the color across the sky above you in the shape of an arc with your palms. Be sure to stretch your arms really wide making a beautiful, broad rainbow arc.
- Repeat this three times.
- Once finished, open your eyes and look up at the beautiful rainbow you and your friends created together.
- Take turns moving around the circle pointing out and sharing which color you contributed to the rainbow.

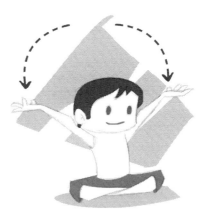

EXHALE

Breathing Techniques

Introduction: *Breathing Techniques*

It is quite natural to not think about or notice our breath, yet the breath can be a very helpful tool – especially when stress, tension or pain are experienced. During periods of stress, the sympathetic nervous system is activated. This is an instinctive and natural human response commonly referred to as "flight or fight" mode and it is activated when a potential threat or danger is sensed. The problem is, it can be–*and often is*— activated when no threat is present.

A variety of stressors can trigger this response and the results range from feelings of tension or anxiety, to rapid or strained breathing, or holding the breath. By learning to recognize these "symptoms" one can consciously turn off these alarm signals by activating the parasympathetic nervous system, ultimately calming the body and mind. The key to activating the parasympathetic nervous system is the breath.

Practicing Breathing Techniques on a regular basis trains the mind and body to respond calmly to stress, anxiety or feelings of discomfort. Additionally, Breathing Techniques develop meditation skills and teach present moment awareness. Calming and relaxing, they can also aid sleeplessness or restlessness, while other exercises are energizing and introduce gentle, fluid body movements. Balancing the brain and the body, Breathing Techniques, provide an excellent mini-break in a child's day allowing them to re-center and refocus, while preparing them to learn and be more productive.

The following chapter introduces twenty-three Breathing Techniques that have been adapted for children of all ages. Practicing these exercises, children will gain an understanding of how their breath works, learn to recognize their own stress triggers, and develop the coping skills necessary to process and regulate reactions and emotions.

Learn. Practice. Breathe. Chill.

Guidelines

- Breath work should always be approached with a sense of ease and gentleness.
- If feelings of discomfort, or shortness of breath are experienced, STOP practicing immediately and recommence regular breathing.
- Never force the breath or create tension within the body.
- Slowly build each practice by incrementally increasing the number of rounds completed, and the depth or length of inhales, exhales and holds.

- Forget how many rounds you completed or how long you practiced yesterday. Approach each practice as if you were doing the exercise for the first time. Start slow and incrementally build to your comfort level.
- Be very mindful to convey this to children who tend to be a little overzealous when initially learning breathing exercises. Foster an understanding of "doing" without "trying" and revert to *Breath Play* activities such as *Bubbles* or *Bubbles in Milk* to demonstrate the sensation of elongating and smoothing the breath without forcing it.

Stress Test

What is Stress Test and how does it help me?

In moments of stress or anxiety we often hold our breath and tense up our entire body without even realizing it. Stress Test demonstrates this in action, teaching us to be aware of this response and how we can change it by consciously relaxing our bodies and controlling our breath.

What will I need?

(Any one of the following)

- Soft rubber or fabric stress ball
- Wad of balled up tissue paper
- Pair of balled up socks

How do I do it?

- You will need one of the props listed above.
- Squeeze it in your fist as tightly as you can for ten seconds. Squeeze really, really tight for the whole ten seconds!
- What happens to your breath? Your shoulders? Other areas of your body?
- Now do the same, but consciously breathe slowly and deeply as you squeeze the prop.
- Scan your body and consciously relax any areas, other than the fist holding and squeezing the prop, where you are tensing up.
- Can you squeeze the prop as tightly as possible while breathing deeply *and* consciously relaxing the rest of your body? It takes a little effort, but it is possible.
- Notice how different this feels to the first try when you most likely held your breath and tensed up your entire body.

No props? No problem!

Tense up your fists and squeeze them as tightly as you can for a count of ten.

Elevator Ride

What is Elevator Ride?

Elevator Ride is a breathing technique that uses creative visualization to teach deep breathing skills while promoting excellent posture.

How does it help me?

Focusing on the spine and the breath together in this exercise encourages the improvement of general posture. Good posture is healthy for your skeletal and muscular systems, it also allows space in the torso for better quality and deeper breathing on a daily basis. Visualizing the breath as a moving object in this exercise is helpful in slowing the breath down, aiding relaxation.

How do I do it?

- Begin in a comfortable seated position. Either crisscross or kneeling with the butt resting on the heels. Use props as needed for support and comfort.
- Rest your hands on top of the thighs and gently close your eyes. Be sure the shoulders are relaxed.
- Gently press your sit bones down, allowing the spine float to a naturally erect position.
- Visualize your spine, running from your tailbone all the way to your skull. Now imagine that your spine is an elevator shaft, with an elevator cab that travels up and down your spine.
- Connecting with your next "IN" breath, feel the elevator rise from your tailbone, all the way to the top floor – Your Head.
- As you breathe "OUT" feel the elevator travel back down the spine, all of the way to the basement – Your Tailbone.
- Continue breathing this way for several rounds using the following visualizations as you do:
    1. Feel the spine grow light and tall as the elevator rises to top floor on your inhale.
    2. Feel grounded and stable as the elevator lowers to the basement on your exhale.
    3. Breathing in, feel the spine grow tall as the elevator travels up your spine to the top floor. Breathing out, feel the elevator as it travels back down the spine – imagine it taking any unwanted feelings, worries, or concerns with it as it lowers down. Imagine these feelings getting off the elevator before you next inhale.
- Continue with elevator breath for 3-5 minutes. Return to normal breathing but remain sitting with the eyes closed for a few more minutes, notice how centered and relaxed you feel.

Belly Breathing

What is Belly Breathing?

Belly breathing, or diaphragmatic breathing, is a deep breathing technique used to relax the mind and body, easing physical and mental tension or stress.

How do I do it?

- Lie in a comfortable position on your yoga mat. As you slowly breathe in, be very conscious of filling your lungs all of the way, when the lungs expand to capacity the belly will raise.
- As you breathe out, be sure to fully empty your lungs, pull your belly button all of the way in, as if your belly button could touch your spine! (This won't really happen, but it is a good visual to help you fully expel all of the air).
- Repeat for several rounds, until you feel calm and relaxed.

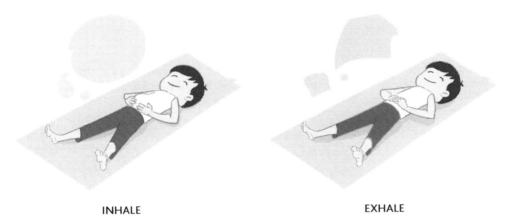

INHALE   EXHALE

Note: Belly breathing may feel weird at first, especially if you are not used to breathing slowly and deeply, or focusing your attention on your breath. With practice it will get easier and feel less strange, and once you enjoy the benefits it will become natural to begin belly breathing any time you need to relax your mind or body.

*Tip: Place your hands, a beanbag, book, or even a toy (such as a rubber-ducky) on your belly to help you observe the effects of your deep belly breathing.

Back Breathing

What is Back Breathing?

Back Breathing is exactly as it sounds, a breathing technique where the focus is on directing the breath into the back area of the body.

How does it help me?

When we breathe in, our chest expands to accommodate the expansion of the lungs as they fill with air. The problem is, we usually do not breathe as fully or deeply as we have the capacity to and the chest barely moves! Back Breathing technique explores breathing fully and deeply by expanding the chest in all directions allowing the lungs to take in more oxygen. Try it for a few minutes several times a day and notice how different you feel!

How do I do it?

- Begin in a comfortable seated position, spine naturally erect, both feet in contact with the floor if siting on a chair. Relax the shoulders and allow your hands to rest in your lap.
- Close your eyes and begin to reflect inwardly, that is, begin to let go of what is happening around you and focus on the inside of your body and mind.
- Begin to observe the breath, don't change it, simply observe as you naturally breathe in and out.
- When you feel ready, slowly begin to deepen the breath.
- After a few rounds of deep breathing, direct your focus to your back.
- On your next inhale visualize the breath "filling" up your entire back. Continue breathing this way for several rounds, noticing how the back spreads and expands with each inhale, and relaxes with each exhale. Imagine your shoulder blades spreading like giant wings as you inhale and relaxing as you exhale.
- Return to natural breathing and gently open the eyes. Notice how your body feels. Notice how your mind feels.

*Tip: Try sitting with your back against a wall. Feel the back expand and press into the wall as you inhale, and relax away from it as you exhale.

PARTNER FUN! Sit back to back with a friend and begin to practice Back Breathing. See if you can feel each other breathe through your backs. Synchronize your breath with your partner's breath and then alternate breaths with your partner, noticing how different each feels.

Side Breathing

What is Side Breathing?

Side Breathing is exactly as it sounds, a breathing technique where the focus is on directing the breath into the side areas of the torso.

How does it help me?

As we breathe in, the chest is designed to expand in all directions to accommodate the expansion of the lungs as they fill with air. The problem is, we usually do not breathe as fully or deeply as we have the capacity to. Side Breathing technique is another fun way of exploring how to breathe fully and deeply. Combined with the techniques *Belly Breathing* and *Back Breathing* we can really learn how different it feels to take full, deep breaths. Try it for a few minutes several times a day and notice how good you feel!

How do I do it?

- Lie on your side and prop your head on a pillow, or on bent elbow/hand.
- Place your other hand on the outer ribs that are facing the ceiling. Clasp the outer rib cage between your thumb and fingers.
- Begin to breathe deeply, until you feel the ribs expanding into the grip of your hand.
- Exhale and observe the ribs retract under your hand.
- Breathe deeply for several rounds, then flip and try it on the other side.
- Once finished, relax for a few moments and notice how you feel.
- Are you naturally breathing deeper than you were before you tried this exercise?

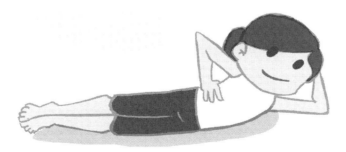

Side Breathing

Sandbag

What is Sandbag?

Sandbag is a breathing technique that uses a sandbag to encourage the body to exhale fully, promoting a deeper sense of relaxation.

How does it help me?

Sandbag is a restorative technique requiring very little muscle engagement or effort to practice. This in itself makes it very relaxing, and the use of the sandbag helps to deepen and slow the breath, further promoting feelings of relaxation while easing feelings of stress or anxiety.

What do I need?

- Small sandbag (DOES NOT need to heavy, a small amount of weight is enough to add resistance).

How do I do it?

- Begin in a comfortable position resting on your back.
- Allow the feet fall open, and the whole body to relax, fully supported by the floor.
- Place a sandbag on your abdomen and begin to inhale. Notice the resistance as your belly presses against the sandbag.
- Exhale slowly, as you complete your exhale, notice how the weight of the sandbag helps you to contract your belly more than usual, allowing a fuller exhale to occur.
- Breathe slowly and deeply for several minutes with the sandbag on your belly.

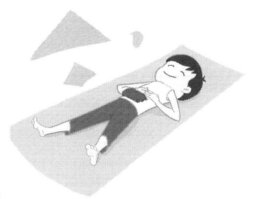

Sandbag

- Remove the sandbag and notice if your breathing pattern changes? Are you still exhaling as fully as you did when you felt the slight weight of the sandbag on your belly? Notice how relaxed you feel after just a few minutes of breathing slowly and deeply.

No sandbag? No problem!

Use a small bag of sugar, flour or rice.

Sun Breath

What is Sun Breath?

Sun Breath is an energizing breath exercise.

How does it help me?

Energizing breath exercises such as Sun Breath can wake you up and give you a little energy when feeling groggy. They can also be a fun way to release any tension or excess energy you may have, Sun Breath is especially good for releasing tension in the jaw and mouth area – common areas people carry tension without being aware of it!

How do I do it?

- Begin standing comfortably with the feet about hip width distance apart.
- Inhale through your nose as you reach your hands toward the sky, as if you were going to grab hold of the sun with both hands.
- Quickly pull your hands back toward you, palms flat facing the middle of your torso as you open your mouth and exhale making a "Ha!" sound. Imagine you are pulling the energy and power of the sun into your own core, or power center.
- Practice for a few rounds.
- Observe how you feel. Do you feel more energized? Do you feel bright and happy like the sun?

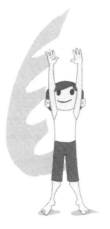

INHALE

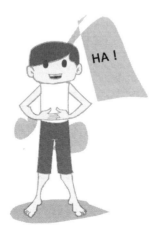

HA !

EXHALE

Sunshine Breath

What is Sunshine Breath?

Sunshine Breath is an active breath exercise linking gentle body movements to your breath cycle.

How does it help me?

By connecting movement to breath you learn about your own breath cycle, and can work toward slowing and controlling it. The physical movement in Sunshine Breath allows more space in the torso to encourage fuller and deeper breaths, calming the nervous system, body and mind. Sunshine Breath can be used as a centering exercise and is excellent to practice before doing something that needs your full attention like meditation, a test or a class.

How do I do it?

Sunshine Breath can be practiced standing, or seated on the floor or in a chair.

Standing: Stand up straight with both feet planted on the ground about hip width distance apart. Slide the shoulder blades down your back and relax arms by your torso.

Floor: Sit comfortably either in crisscross or kneeling. Spine naturally erect, shoulders relaxed and arms resting by torso.

Chair: Sit comfortably with both feet planted on the floor, spine naturally erect, and shoulders relaxed with the arms resting by torso.

- Gently close your eyes, or softly gaze at a point in front of you.
- Turn your attention inward and begin to observe your natural breath as it flows in and out for a few rounds.
- On an inhale sweep the arms up in a big circle until the palms meet high above your head.
- Exhale, keeping the palms pressed together, draw them down toward the middle of your chest, or heart.
- Inhale, keep the palms pressed together and straighten the arms back up overhead.
- Exhale circle the arms back down along side the torso. This is one complete round. Repeat 3-5 full rounds.
- Sit quietly and enjoy the sensations created by this movement and deep breathing.

*Tip: Remember to link the movement to your breath, make each movement match your inhale and exhale. Like a car does not move without gas, your body should not move without an "in" or "out" breath fueling it.

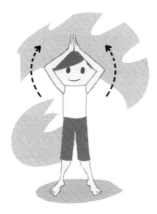

INHALE

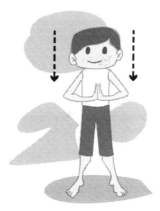

EXHALE

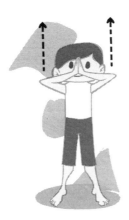

INHALE

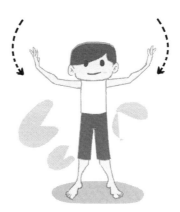

EXHALE

Centering

What is Centering?

Centering is a technique that connects the mind and body, resulting in an immediate sense of calm and relaxation. Centering can be used in preparation to focus on an activity such as meditation, speaking, or an important class or exam.

How does it help me?

Centering stops the chatter of the mind, bringing us to the present moment. Eliminating distractions and promoting awareness, Centering empowers us to be calm, focused and ready for anything.

How do I do it?

- Begin sitting comfortably on the floor or in a chair, or standing with the feet hip width apart. Spine naturally erect, arms, shoulders and face relaxed.
- Inhale deeply as you sweep your arms out to the side and up overhead bringing the palms to touch.
- Keep the palms pressed together and slowly slide them toward your heart as you exhale.
- Repeat for several rounds until you feel calm, relaxed and centered.

*Tip: Each movement should last as long as each inhale or exhale. Kind of like gas in a car, without gas the car does not move, but if there is gas, the car moves. Likewise, your body should only move when you are either inhaling or exhaling – no breath, no movement.

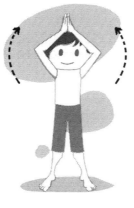

INHALE

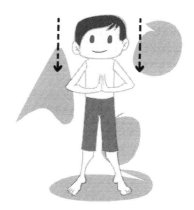

EXHALE

Equal Breath

What is Equal Breath?

Equal Breath is exactly as it sounds, an exercise where you control your breath by breathing in and out to an equal count.

How does it help me?

Equal Breath relaxes the body while fully engaging the mind, making it an excellent exercise in concentration or focus. Use this exercise to relax during moments of stress, to refocus before an important class, or to help quiet the mind and relax the body if you are experiencing insomnia.

How do I do it?

- Begin in a comfortable position either seated or lying on your back.
- Close your eyes and turn your attention inward.
- Shift your attention to your breath. DO NOT change anything about your breath, just let it flow in and out naturally, observing it as it does so.
- As you breathe in count in your mind, 1-2-3.
- As you breathe out count in your mind 1-2-3.
- Once you complete several rounds, and it feels comfortable, increase the count.
- As you breathe in, count in your mind 1-2-3-4.
- As your breathe out, count in your mind 1-2-3-4.
- Once you complete several rounds, scan the body and see if you are holding tension anywhere. If you still feel relaxed, try adding an extra count for a few rounds (e.g. 1-2-3-4-5). If breathing this way has created tension somewhere in your body or mind, relax and go back to a lower count, 1-2-3.

*Tips:

- Always check in with your body as you practice this exercise, treat each time you approach it as a new, and be sure you stay relaxed and are not creating tension by forcing a higher count.
- Slowly build the count and always drop back to a lower count if you notice any signs of tension in the body, mind or the breath.
- You WILL experience the effects of this exercise with a lower count, you WILL NOT experience any positive effects from this exercise if you force through to a higher count, creating tension in the body and mind.

Fuel Your Moves

What is Fuel Your Moves?

Fuel Your Moves is an exercise where you do exactly that – Fuel Your Moves, by connecting each movement to either an "in" or "out" breath.

How does it help me?

Connecting movement to breath does two things: It slows the breath down resulting in feelings of relaxation, and it links the mind to the physical body, a form meditation and present moment awareness that promotes calmness and an ability to focus. The gentle physical movements shown in Fuel Your Moves are great tension relievers and provide a mini-break for the mind and body after using a computer or sitting for long periods of time.

How do I do it?

- Begin sitting comfortably on the floor or in a chair, or standing, feet hip width apart. Spine should be naturally erect, arms and shoulders relaxed.
- Linking each of your inhales and exhales to a movement, follow the guide below repeating each move for a total of 3-5 full rounds before moving to the next.
- Remember! Each movement should last for the duration of each inhale or exhale. Gas fuels a car to move, and your breath is what fuels your body to move in this exercise - no breath, no movement!

Shoulder Shrugs

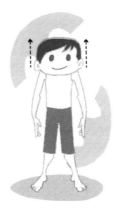   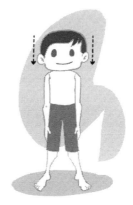

INHALE   EXHALE

Inhale – Lift shoulders up toward the ears.

Exhale – Lower shoulders, sliding blades down the back.

Repeat 3-5 times.

Shoulder Rolls

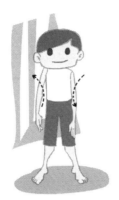
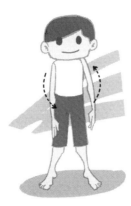

INHALE   EXHALE

Inhale – Roll right shoulder forward and up toward ear. At the same time, drop left shoulder back and down.

Exhale – Roll left shoulder forward and up toward ear, at the same time drop the right shoulder back and down.

Switch directions, completing 3-5 rounds in each direction.

Chin Drop

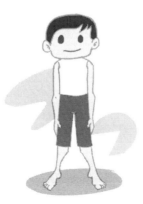
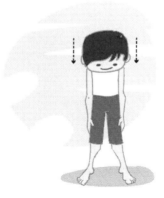

INHALE   EXHALE

Inhale – Look straight ahead keeping chin level with the floor.

Exhale – Drop chin toward chest, stretching the back of the neck.

Repeat 3-5 times.

Neck Rolls

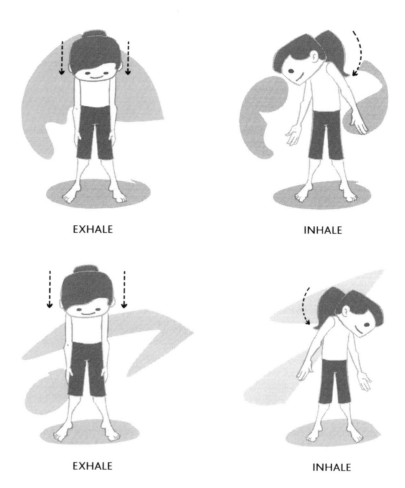

EXHALE   INHALE

EXHALE   INHALE

Inhale – Look straight ahead keeping chin level with the floor.

Exhale – Drop chin to chest.

Inhale – Keeping chin close to the chest, roll chin toward right shoulder.

Exhale – Keeping chin close to the chest, roll chin back to center.

Inhale – Keeping chin close to the chest, roll chin to left shoulder.

Keep the chin close to the chest, and repeat 3-5 times. Once complete, roll chin to center of chest and inhale as you float the head up to a neutral position, chin level with the floor.

Gentle Twists

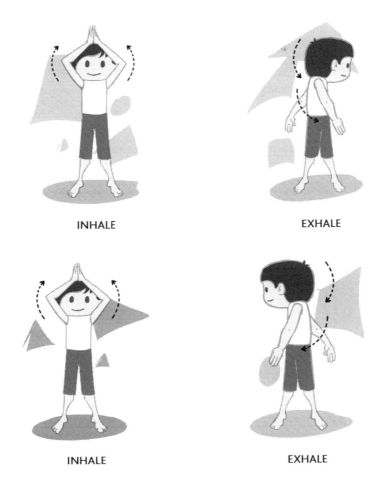

Inhale – Sweep the arms up overhead.

Exhale – Lowering arms, gently twist to the left, keep hips facing front as you twist the torso, shoulders and head to the left.

Inhale – Return to center, sweeping arms back overhead.

Exhale – Lowering arms, gently twist to the right, keep hips facing front as you twist the torso, shoulders and head to the right.

Repeat 3-5 times.

Three-Part Breath

What is Three-Part Breath?

Three-Part Breath is a breathing technique that demonstrates how to breathe deeply and fully.

How does it help me?

Three-Part Breath slows your breathing down and steadies it, promoting a sense of calm, relaxation and control. Three-Part Breath teaches how to utilize the full breathing system you were born with, encouraging full and deep inhales rather than the short and shallow breaths we usually get by with.

How do I do it?

- Sit comfortably in a chair, spine naturally erect, shoulders relaxed with hands resting on knees or thighs, and both feet flat on the floor.
- Gently place one hand on the upper chest area below the collarbones, and one hand on the belly. Be sure to keep the shoulders and arms relaxed as you rest the hands on these two areas.
- Take a deep, slow breath in through your nose, filling the lower part of your lungs – you should feel your belly pressing against your hand as this happens.
- Slowly breathe out, feeling your belly retract as you do. Imagine you are pulling your belly button in to touch your spine – this will help fully expel all of the air.
- Breathe in and out this way for five full breaths.
- After five breaths, breathe in once again, this time filling up the lungs until the belly presses against your hand, and then sip in a little more air, filling up the chest. Notice the ribs and breastbone expand as the middle of your torso fills with the extra breath.
- As you exhale, feel the ribs relax as the air from your middle releases first, followed by the belly button moving toward the spine as the air expels from the belly.
- Repeat deep breathing into the belly and the ribcage for five full breaths.
- After five breaths, breathe in again, this time filling up the belly, followed by the ribcage, and then, fill the upper-chest cavity with more air so that you feel your collarbones spreading, almost like they are breaking into a huge smile.
- Exhale, first emptying the upper chest so that the collarbones relax, then the middle chest and finally the belly. Pulling the belly button all the way toward the spine, fully expelling all of the air.

- Continue to breathe this way for five full breaths.
- You are now practicing Three-Part Breath. As you practice, work toward making the three-parts one smooth movement rather than breaking it up with pauses. It will still be Three-Part Breath – filling the lower lungs, the middle and then the top – in one long breath, without pauses. The exhale will be the same – first emptying the upper lungs, the middle and finally, the lower, in one long exhale.
- Repeat for 5-10 rounds.

*Tip: Three-Part Breathing can be practiced while lying in bed! It can slow down your mind if you are thinking a lot and help you sleep better.

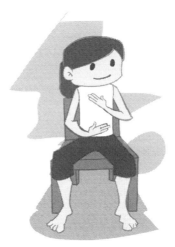

Three-Part Breath

Lengthening the Exhale

What is Lengthening the Exhale and how does it help me?

When you exhale your body relaxes, it also physically "lets go", releasing converted CO_2 gases that your body does not need. Lengthening the Exhale cultivates a deeper sense of release and relaxation within the body and the mind; it also slows the breath down, which calms the nervous system and relieves feelings of stress or anxiety as well as physical tension.

How do I do it?

- Begin in a comfortable position, either seated on the floor or in a chair, or lying down with the knees bent and feet flat on the floor.
- Shift your focus to the natural breath. Observing it in its natural state for a few rounds.
- Begin to deepen and slow the breath.
- Count your inhale and your exhale and work toward making them last for the same number of counts. For example, Inhale 1-2-3 and Exhale 1-2-3
- Following several rounds of breathing with an equal inhale and exhale, begin to slow your exhale down even more until it is several counts slower than the inhale. For example, Inhale 1-2-3, exhale 1-2-3-4
- Be sure to exhale fully each time before breathing in again.
- NEVER take the inhale-to-exhale ratio beyond 1:2 (i.e. never exhale for a count greater than double your inhale count).
- Be creative and visualize stress or tension leaving your body each time you exhale.

*Tip: Take it beyond the physical:

When we breathe in, we breathe in fresh oxygen, which our body needs. When we breathe out, we eliminate waste from our body, which has been converted to carbon dioxide. When we breathe in, our lungs expand and our diaphragm contracts, and when we breathe out, our diaphragm and lungs relax.

Essentially, when we breathe in, we are expanding and filling ourselves up with what we need, and when we breathe out, we are letting go of stuff we don't need or is no longer useful, and we are relaxing. Use your imagination and visualize letting go of any thoughts or feelings that hold you back as you exhale – it can be anything from anger to jealousy to self-doubt, allow these feelings to leave with each exhale.

4 Square Breathing

What is 4 Square Breathing?

Breathing is something we do naturally without thinking too much about it. If we were to describe how we breathe, we would most likely say that we breathe in and out in two simple steps. But, there are actually four steps to each breath we take:

1. Inhale
2. Pause
3. Exhale
4. Pause

4-Square-Breathing is a technique used to emphasize each stage of the breath, slowing it down and calming the mind, body and nervous system.

How does it help me?

A very effective relaxation tool, this technique is extremely helpful in alleviating anxiety and stress and can be used to center yourself before a test, or any situation where you want to feel calm, centered and focused.

How do I do it?

- Begin in a comfortable seated position, spine naturally erect and chin level. Be sure that your shoulders, arms and face relaxed. Hands should rest comfortably in your lap, or on the knees.
- Observe your natural breath cycle for a few rounds before beginning to deepen the breath.
- Breathe all the way in until your belly expands, and then all the way out until the belly button moves toward the spine, expelling all of the air.
- When you feel ready to begin, inhale to a count of THREE.
- Once inhale is complete, hold the breath in for a count of TWO.
- Slowly exhale, with control, for a count of THREE.
- Hold all of the air OUT for a count of TWO.
- Continue breathing this way for 3-5 full rounds.

*Tip: As you practice and become more comfortable with this breathing technique, incrementally build up to 10 full rounds with a count of FOUR for each stage – Inhale for FOUR, Hold for FOUR, Exhale for FOUR, and Hold out for FOUR. NEVER go higher than four counts for each stage of the breath AND you MUST take your time and BUILD VERY SLOWLY to this level when *your* body is ready (not your mind!).

Take Five

What is Take Five?

Take Five is a breathing technique that acts as a quick fix, helping us to breathe and relax, especially during moments of stress. Take Five is common expression used when people intend to take a break from a task or job they are doing, in this instance think of it as a break for your mind and body. You can "Take Five" anytime you feel you need it.

How does it help me?

When we feel nervous, anxious or stressed a very natural reaction is to hold the breath, breathe rapidly, or breathe in uneven and choppy bursts. These reactions only create more stress within the mind and body. Take Five teaches us to connect with the breath and use it as a tool to steady and calm the mind and body. Sometimes we cannot change or control a situation or experience but we can control how we react to it. The ability to slow and even out the breath is a fantastic tool to have in your toolbox; it enables you to take control of how you respond to stress and tension.

How do I do it?

- Hold your hand up, splaying all four fingers and the thumb wide.
- Slowly breathe in to the count of five, curling one finger in at a time as you count off 1-2-3-4-5.
- Once you reach five, pause, and then slowly breath out to a count of five, extending one finger at a time back out as you count, 1-2-3-4-5.
- Repeat for several rounds.
- Return to natural breathing.
- Check in with your natural breath rhythm – you should find it is naturally slower and more even after completing just a few rounds of Take Five.
- Check in with how you feel – you should feel a lot more centered and calm.

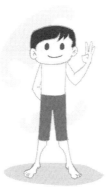

Take Five Breathing

Big Round Tire Breath

What is Big Round Tire Breath and how does it help me?

Big Round Tire Breath is an exercise that focuses on letting go and releasing. Slowing the breath down, this exercise is very calming to the mind and body. Try it for several rounds and notice how different you feel.

How do I do it?

Begin in a comfortable seated position:

- Sit comfortably in a chair, spine naturally erect, shoulders relaxed, hands resting on thighs and feet flat on the floor.
- Take a deep breath in through your nose, filling up your entire torso—like a big round tire—with air.
- Pause and then slowly release the air through your teeth making a hissing sound, like a tire with a slow, steady leak.
- As you let the "air" slowly hiss out of your body, imagine any negative thoughts, fears, worries, or emotions leaving with it.
- Repeat for 3-5 rounds

*Tip: Big Round Tire Breath can be practiced anywhere – even when you have to wait in a long line at the movies.

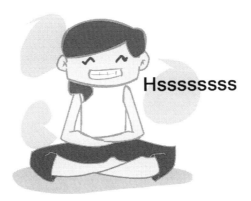

Big Round Tire Breath

Alternate Nostril Breathing

What is Alternate Nostril Breathing and how does it help me?

Practicing Alternate Nostril Breathing helps to balance the two hemispheres of the brain. It aids in slowing the breath down, calming the nervous system, and relieving stress and anxiety. This breathing exercise is excellent for insomnia.

How do I do it?

- Begin in a comfortable upright position, either seated on the floor in crisscross or kneeling, or in a chair. Spine naturally erect, but relaxed.
- Rest your left hand in your lap and raise your right hand toward your face. Gently close off your right nostril by lightly pressing the outside of it with your thumb.
- Inhale through your left nostril, and then close left nostril by lightly pressing it with your ring and little fingers.
- Release the thumb from the right nostril and exhale slowly and fully through the right nostril.
- Keeping the right nostril open, inhale fully, and then close it off with the thumb.
- Release the ring and little fingers from left nostril and exhale slowly and fully out of the left nostril. This completes one cycle. Repeat 3 to 5 times.
- Release hand to rest in the lap and commence normal breathing. Sit with the eyes closed enjoying the sensations of balance and serenity this exercise brings.

*Tips:

- Be sure to keep shoulders relaxed. If the arms become fatigued, use both hands and alternate blocking each nostril with the index finger of each hand.
- If you are left-hand dominant, reverse this exercise using your left hand and begin by blocking off the left nostril with the thumb and the right nostril with the ring and pinkie fingers.

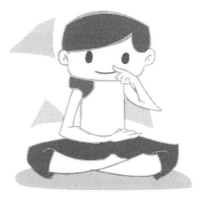

Alternate Nostril Breathing

Taco Tongue

What is Taco Tongue?

While it certainly sounds silly, Taco Tongue is a breathing technique that has a cooling and calming effect on the body and nervous system. The long sides of the tongue are curled in to form a taco-like shape, hence, the name Taco Tongue.

How does it help me?

Think of a puppy panting when he is playing, this is his way of cooling his body when it begins to warm from activity – by drawing cool air over his tongue, his body begins to cool. When you practice Taco-Tongue breathing, you create a straw or tube like shape with your tongue and draw air over its surface, cooling the tongue and the body. Taco-Tongue also triggers a calming response in the nervous system – reducing negative mind/body states such as anxiety or anger. Excellent for developing focus and concentration, if you practice Taco-Tongue several times daily you'll be sharp, attentive, and cool as a cucumber… or should that be an avocado?

How do I do it?

- Begin in a comfortable seated position, spine naturally erect, shoulders, arms, and face relaxed, hands resting in the lap.
- *Curl both sides of the tongue inwardly, rolling it into a straw shape, like a taco.
- Slowly breathe in through the straw-like shape your tongue has formed.
- Once your inhale is complete, draw the tongue back into your mouth and relax it (allow it to unroll) as you exhale slowly through the nose.
- Repeat.
- As you practice Taco-Tongue gradually build to 8-12 rounds per sitting.

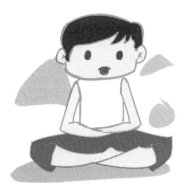

Taco Tongue

*Tip: If you are unable to curl your tongue lengthwise (it's okay, many people are anatomically unable to do this) try the following:

- Relax the jaw, allowing the mouth to drop open slightly.
- Rest the tip of the tongue behind the upper teeth.
- Inhale slowly through the space between the teeth.
- Once inhale is complete, relax the tongue and close the mouth and exhale through the nose. Repeat, building to 8-12 rounds per sitting.

Darth Vader/Ocean Breath

What is Darth Vader or Ocean Breath?

Darth Vader or Ocean Breath is a loud and rhythmic breathing technique. Connecting to the sound and rhythm of the breath using this method has two advantages: It can be used as a focal point in meditation to direct our minds to the present moment. It can also be used as a gauge during physical activity, observing the smoothness and evenness of the breath in response to any movements we make with the physical body. (Bearing in mind that when we are over-stressing the body, the breath becomes choppy or strained, a sign that we should scale back whatever we are doing until the breath sounds smooth, even and unstressed once again.)

How does it help me?

Darth Vader or Ocean Breath really does sound like the Star Wars character or the ocean; focusing on the breath and the sound it creates improves concentration and calms and focuses the mind. This technique is effective for calming the nervous system, reducing pain, and aiding insomnia and headaches.

How do I do it?

- Begin in a comfortable seated position. Sit up tall, yet relaxed.
- Take a slow inhale through the nose.
- Open the mouth and exhale with an "aaaaaaaah" sound.
- Repeat 2-3 times.
- Inhale through the nose, then, keeping the mouth closed, exhale as if making the "aaaah" sound, only the mouth remains closed this time.
- You should hear your breath make a soft "hissing" sound – like Darth Vader from Star Wars or the ocean.
- Continue to breath this way, breathing in and out through the nose with the mouth closed… making the gentle hissing sound as if you were breathing out of the mouth saying "aaaaaaaah".
- Keep breathing this way for several rounds. You may notice that your throat is slightly constricted to create this sound– not strongly or tightly, just enough to create the gentle rhythmic sound. The breath should remain smooth and controlled, not strained or forced.
- Build up slowly, taking breaks in between to breath naturally. At first it may feel weird, but as you practice you will be able to breathe this way for longer periods.
- Gently place your fingers in your ears, and focus on the sound of the breath within your body.
- Have fun with it – pretend you are in your very own Star Wars movie, or, imagine the soothing and rhythmic ocean within you, vast, powerful and strong.

Breathe In, Breathe Out, Chillax

What is Breathe In, Breathe Out, Chillax?

Breathe In, Breathe Out, Chillax is a simple mantra-type breathing exercise you can practice anywhere and any time. This technique serves as a quick fix during moments of tension, stress or anxiety, as well as to calm oneself when excess energy or silliness bubbles within.

How does it help me?

Immediately drawing attention to your breath, Breathe In, Breathe Out, Chillax, is a breathing technique that encourages slow and steady breathing, calming the nervous system and disarming the fight or flight response – a natural reaction to stressful situations. Breathe In, Breathe Out, Chillax is a handy tool you can access any time you need it, the simple mantra keeps you connected to the breath and what you are doing, removing the focus from anything that may have triggered feelings of stress, anxiety, or worry.

How do I do it?

- When you find yourself experiencing a moment of stress or anxiety (or impatience waiting in a long line!), immediately draw your attention to your breath.
- Close your mouth and begin to breathe through your nose.
- Slow and deepen your next inhale, saying the words, "Breathe In" to yourself as you feel the ribs expanding in all directions.
- As you breathe out through the nose, slowly and with control, say the words "Breathe Out" to yourself.
- Once the air is expelled, and before taking your next inhale, say the word "Chillax" to yourself.
- Repeat for several rounds until you feel yourself relaxing and taking deeper, slower breaths naturally.

Blow it Away

What is Blow it Away?

Blow it Away is a creative visualization exercise that uses the breath to encourage letting go.

How does it help me?

Blow it Away guides you toward any negative feelings or thought patterns you may be harboring and gives you the opportunity to peacefully let them go. Using the exhale, which is the body letting go of "stuff" it no longer needs (CO_2), you can also let go of non-physical "stuff" such as worries and anxieties.

How do I do it?

- Begin in a comfortable seated position.
- Cup your hands together with the palms facing up to form a bowl.
- Visualize anything that is bugging you or constantly on your mind sitting in the bowl of your hands.
- Take a long inhale through your nose.a
- Exhale by blowing the air into your hands, sending your worry far away. (Experiment with a short, strong exhale, or soft and gentle blowing action – see which feels better for you).
- Sit quietly for a few moments and notice how you feel. Do you feel lighter?

Note: If your worries remain after trying an exercise like this, or keep coming back, it may be a good idea to talk to a parent, trusted teacher or friend about what is on your mind.

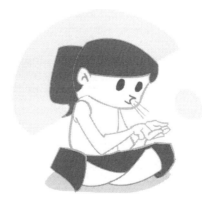

Blow it Away

Dragon Breath

What is Dragon Breath?

Ever wish you could be a fire-breathing dragon? Well, you can! Dragon Breath is a fun way to relax the entire body and mind very quickly.

How does it help me?

Dragon Breath is a great tool if you are feeling stressed, or if you have been working hard physically or mentally and need a break. The releasing, or letting go element of Dragon Breath will have your mind and body feeling calm and relaxed in no time.

How do I do it?

- Begin in a comfortable position, either seated or lying on the floor.
- Alternatively, you can begin in child's pose. Knees bent on the floor, torso resting on top of thighs and forehead resting on floor. Allow the arms to rest on the floor along side the torso, palms facing up.
- Take a deep breath in through the nose, filling the lungs until your belly pushes out.
- Open the mouth and let the air escape with an *"Aaaaaah".
- Repeat 3-5 times.

*Tip: This is not like Lion's Breath where you roar and make a lot of noise forcing the air out. To practice Dragon Breath, open the mouth and let the air flow out softly, like a fire-breathing dragon toasting a soft marsh-mellow. If he forces the air out he will burn the marsh-mellow to a crisp, if he aspirates, the heat from his breath will gently and evenly toast the delicate marsh-mellow to perfection.

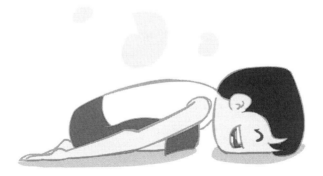

Dragon Breath

Whale Breath

What is Whale Breath and how does it help me?

Whale Breath is a relaxing breath and body movement that releases lower back tension by lengthening and gently rotating the spine. Using the breath and gravity, the spine gently releases into a twist and lengthens as the rest of the body relaxes. Linking movement to breath slows the breath down and deepens it, resulting in deeper levels of relaxation.

How do I do it?

- Lie on your back. Place both feet flat on the floor with the knees pointing up toward the ceiling. Feet can be hip-width distance apart or wider.
- Extend the arms out along the floor in a "t" position. Take a deep breath in through the nose.
- Keep both shoulders pressed into the floor, drop both knees over to the right and turn your head to look left as you slowly blow the air out through your mouth.
- Inhale through the nose as you bring the knees and head back to center; exhale through the mouth as you drop the knees to the left and turn the head to the right.
- Repeat for several rounds.

*Tip: As you twist, it is important that both shoulders stay in contact with the floor. Your knees may not make it all the way to floor, this will happen with time. Eventually gravity, combined with the deep release encouraged by your exhales, will soften any physical resistance and tightness.

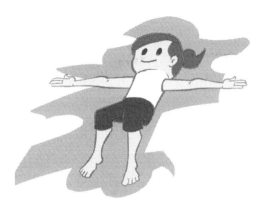

INHALE

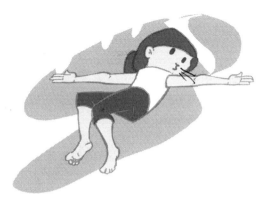

EXHALE

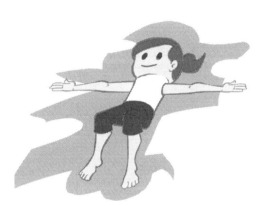

INHALE

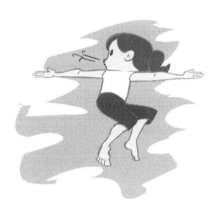

EXHALE

Section 3

Relaxation and Meditation Techniques

Introduction: *Relaxation and Meditation Techniques*

Imagine leaving your smartphone, iPod, computer, or tablet on all of the time and never turning it off or recharging it. Eventually, the battery will burn out. Well, people—*and kids*—are no different! The mind and body are both very busy machines that work incredibly hard and, not unlike a computer or iPod, resting and recharging are key to optimal performance and avoiding burnout.

Lumosity, the popular online brain-fitness program, credits meditation as follows: *"Periodically calming and focusing the mind has been shown to improve processing speed, attention, and response times."*

The exercises presented in the following chapter provide the tools and know-how to consciously relax and revive the body and mind. Removing stimulation and practicing these exercises will provide an opportunity for kids to relax and enjoy the benefits of a mini-break, calming and soothing the body, mind and nervous system. Reemerging with a sense of calm, serenity and wellbeing, children develop an understanding of and appreciation for the value of meditation and relaxation, inspiring them to practice on their own and well into adulthood.

Guidelines

- Before practicing relaxation or meditation techniques, remove any stimuli or potential distractions. Cell phones should be switched off and do not disturb signs hung if appropriate.

- Be sure that everybody is comfortable and has anything they may need within reach – blankets, pillows, eye pillows etc.

- Dim lights and play soft, soothing music as required.

- Kids may fall asleep during a particularly long or relaxing practice. Before commencing, tell them that this may happen, that it is very natural and they should not feel embarrassed if they do. Falling asleep means they needed the rest.

- When rousing a sleeping child, it is very important not to startle or frighten them.

- Use a feather to gently stroke their hands, feet or face. Be sure to explain this is what you will be doing should they fall asleep BEFORE commencing practice and talk to them as you apply the feather strokes. For example, "The magic wake-up feather is gently waking you up now…" etc.

Tap-Tap-Tap

What is Tap-Tap-Tap?

Tap-Tap-Tap is a self-massage technique that not only feels great, but also gets all of the cells in your body buzzing, providing the anchor for a meditation that focuses on sensation.

How does it help me?

Often we "live" inside our heads, or, externally focused on everybody and everything around us, without paying too much attention to our own bodies and minds. Self-massage and meditation help you to be in tune with and understand your body – allowing you to discover any areas where you may be holding tension that you can then work toward relaxing using stretching and breathing techniques or simple awareness. Beyond self-massage, the sensations created when you use the Tap-Tap-Tap technique make a great focal point to sit in a meditation fully absorbing the benefits of your massage, enhancing body awareness and promoting a deep sense relaxation.

How do I do it?

- Begin in a comfortable seated position in a chair or on the floor.
- Using gentle finger pressure, lightly tap the top of your head.
- Move along the back of the head, the sides of the head and temples, and across the forehead.
- Gently tap around the eye sockets, back to the temples and down the jaw.
- Squeeze each shoulder with the opposite hand, like you are kneading dough to make bread.
- Fold your hands into soft fists and gently tap across the chest – you can let some sounds out here like Tarzan pounding his chest.

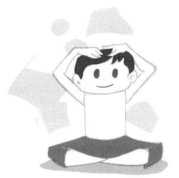

Tap-Tap-Tap

- Gently tap the fist down the inside of one arm, tap the palm and the back of hand, and then tap all the way back up the outside of the arm.
- Tap across the chest again to the opposite arm and repeat.
- With palms flat, gently pat the belly area, then sides of the torso and reach around the back and gently pat the kidney area and lower back.
- Starting at the top of one thigh, gently tap your fist down the inside of the leg, tap the sole of the foot, top of the foot, and all the way back up the outside of the leg. Repeat on the other leg.
- Once finished, gently close the eyes and notice all of the sensations you can feel in the body. Really focus in great detail on each sensation – tingling, buzzing etc. – observing all of the sensations your massage has created until they fade.
- When you feel ready, slowly open your eyes and notice how GOOD you feel.

The Sshh Game

What is The Sshh Game?

The Sshh Game is a fun present moment awareness exercise that is easy for kids of all ages to play.

How does it help me?

Present moment awareness is a great tool to access when you need to focus or concentrate. A form of meditation, it is also helpful if you find yourself caught up in thoughts that are not helpful, or at times when you have trouble falling asleep.

How do I do it?

This game can be played in a group or individually:

Group:

- Begin sitting comfortably in a circle. (Large groups can be broken up into several smaller groups.)
- Center the group by doing a couple of rounds of *Balloon Breath* (*Breathing Techniques*).
- Determine an order or direction for each member of the circle to take his or her turn.
- Each person begins his or her turn by saying "Sshh..." and the rest of the group remains quiet as each person takes their turn. Once each person feels and then acknowledges a sensation, the next person takes their turn.

Individual:

- Begin in a comfortable seated position.
- Close eyes and take a few deep inhales and exhales until you feel centered.

The Sshh Game:

- Sit quietly and wait until you sense something – smell, taste, sound or sensation.
- When you do, say "Sshh...", "I can feel...", or, "I can smell...", or, "I can hear..." etc.
- Sit quietly and wait for the next sensation to arise and acknowledge it.
- For example: "Sshh... I can feel a breeze on my arm"; "Sshh... I can hear a bird singing"; "Sshh... I can feel my own heart beating"; "Sshh.... I can hear a plane flying by" etc.
- Sometimes you may not hear, feel, smell or taste anything – just sit quietly and wait until you do. The more quietly you sit and "Sshh" the more likely you are to notice things.

*Tip: Teachers - the "Sshh" or quiet component necessary to play this game, makes it effective in quieting and calming a class that has become rowdy.

Magic Feather Meditation

What is Magic Feather Meditation?

Magic Feather Meditation is a relaxation technique that uses feathers and light feather strokes to calm and relax the body and mind.

How does it help me?

Light feather strokes sooth and calm the nervous system and gently stimulate the sensory system, helping with body awareness and proprioception (sense of where the physical body is positioned or located in space). Most people find this exercise soothing and relaxing – like magic!

How do I do it?

Magic Feather Meditation is best done partnered up with a friend, however it can be adapted as a self-massage/meditation technique.

Partner Activity:

- One partner lies comfortably on the floor with eyes gently closed. Guide them to relax fully by taking a few deep inhales and exhales before letting go, allowing the breath to be natural and the body to be relaxed, fully supported by the floor.
- The second person, using a feather, gently applies soft strokes along the arms and legs, torso and the face – gently tracing the jawline, temples, forehead, bridge of nose and neck (avoid the inside of the ears and nose, and avoid the eyes).
- Encourage the person applying the feather strokes to also use this exercise as a meditation, staying focused and present, observing any subtle responses in their partner. Switch roles.

Individual Meditation/Self Massage:

Begin in a comfortable seated position. Close your eyes and take a few deep inhales and exhales to feel centered and present. Using a feather, gently begin to apply soft feathery strokes to your body. Try out different pressures and strokes, noticing how it makes you feel and which areas of the body you are drawn to – do you notice you are holding tension in that particular area? OR, follow this simple routine:

- Begin with light feather strokes on the back of the hand and fingers. Move to the palm, then along the arm, all the way to the shoulder (be sure to cover entire arm, back and front with light feathery strokes). Repeat other arm.
- Gently sweep the feather along the jawline, temples, across the forehead and down the bridge of nose. Over the chin, under the chin, and on the neck (be sure to sweep sides and back of neck if your feather can reach).

- Gently sweep across chest and down to the belly. Sweep the sides of the torso to the hips.
- Sweep down one leg all of the way to the foot (be sure to cover entire leg, back and front).
- Sweep the top of the foot and ankle and then the sole of the foot with the feather. Repeat other side.

No feather? No problem!

Use your fingertips! Apply very soft, gentle strokes by lightly dragging your fingertips in an upward or downward motion, barely touching the body.

*Tips:

- Use short, upward strokes to energize, and long, downward strokes to calm.
- Teachers – this is an excellent technique to use to gently awaken a student who falls asleep during a meditation or relaxation practice. Be VERY gentle so as not to startle them, and talk to them softly as you apply light feather strokes. For example, "The magic wake-up feather is gently waking you up now."

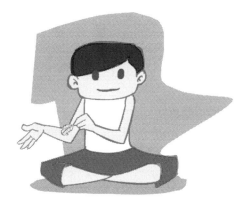

Magic Feather Meditation

Snow Globe Meditation

What is Snow Globe Meditation?

Snow Globe Meditation is a fun craft project that teaches how to settle or quiet down the mind when it is too busy or overwhelmed with a lot of thoughts and/or feelings.

How does it help me?

People are very busy and we often have many things on our minds. Sometimes we have so many thoughts swirling around all at once that we cannot begin to think straight. Not only is this overwhelming and exhausting, but unhealthy for the mind and the body. Meditation can help by quieting the mind, giving it a rest so to speak. Learning to meditate and introducing regular meditation practice helps to clear the mind and alleviate feelings of stress or anxiety.

What do I need?

1 Small Glass Jar with Lid (Rinse an old jelly, infant food or mason jar)

Glitter (Several colors if possible)

Liquid Glycerin

Liquid hand or dish soap (Clear if possible)

How do I do it?

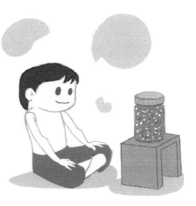

Snow Globe Meditation

- Fill clean, glass jar ¾ full with warm tap water.
- Adding liquid glycerin, fill to about ¼ inch from top.
- Add 3-4 drops of liquid soap.
- Tighten the lid on jar and gently agitate until liquids mix together.
- The clear fluid in the jar is like your mind in its clear, natural state. Place the jar in front of you and remove the lid. Take a moment to observe your mind for a moment, as a thought arises place a pinch of glitter in the jar to represent that thought. You can use a different color glitter (if you have it) for each thought or for the type of thought you are having (e.g. sad, angry, scared, etc.). Once you feel ready, place the lid firmly back on the jar and give it a shake. Watch all of your "thoughts" swirl around in the jar… isn't that just how your mind feels sometimes?
- Settle the jar on a flat surface in front of you and sit comfortably and quietly. Begin to breathe in and out slowly as you watch the glitter slowly settle toward the bottom of the jar. As the glitter slows down and settles, allow your thoughts to do the same.

*Tip: Keep your jar and use it whenever you feel overwhelmed by thoughts, or when you simply need to clear your mind and relax.

Scarves

What is Scarves and how does it help me?

Scarves is a fun mirroring game that can be played in partners or groups. An active meditation, it encourages slow, fluid physical movements and a quiet, focused mind to play. In addition to the benefits of meditation—a clear, calm and focused mind—Scarves develops coordination skills and balance, while fostering teamwork and intuition.

What do I need?

- One colorful silk scarf per child.

How do I do it?

- Begin in partners facing each other, one child elected as leader. Or in small groups with one child facing each group as the leader.
- The leader slowly moves his scarf around in slow and fluid movements. His partner or group must follow, mirroring his moves.
- Can you match the leader's movements? Can you match the leader's speed?
- Leaders are encouraged to keep movements slow and intentional, this is more challenging to mirror than fast, jerky movements and requires a lot more presence.

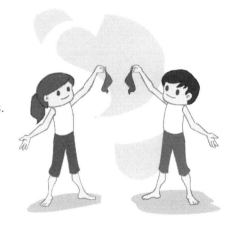

Scarves

- After working with the same leader for a while, do you notice that you begin to guess what their next move will be, naturally moving with them without thinking too much about it? This is your intuition.

Discussion: After playing scarves begin an open discussion with players about how they felt in their minds while playing. Did they find it easy to focus on the scarf and the leader's moves? Or were they easily distracted? Did any players experience their intuition coming into play? If so, discuss intuition – what it is and how it can play a role in other areas of their lives.

Game: Scarves can be played as a game of elimination: The child "caught" not mirroring the move exactly is "it" - in the case of a group activity, one player will be eliminated from each round until only one player remains and is declared the winner. In the case of a partner activity, the person who is not "it" gets a point, roles are switched and the game begins again. Whoever has the most points at the end is the Mirror Champion.

Pencils

What is Pencils and how does it help me?

Pencils is a fun game to play with a friend or partner anytime! An active meditation, it encourages a quiet, focused mind to play. In addition to the benefits of meditation –a clear, calm and focused mind– Pencils develops coordination skills while fostering trust and teamwork.

What will I need?

- Two new pencils – unsharpened (flat on both ends)

How do I do it?

- Begin in a comfortable seated position facing your partner.
- Hold one palm up to face your partner's palm, like a mirror. For example, if partner A holds up his left palm, partner B would hold up his right palm.
- Place one pencil between the palms. Gently press palms into the flat end of the pencil, suspending the pencil in the air between each partner's palms.
- Begin to move the pencil around without dropping it.
- Take turns leading.

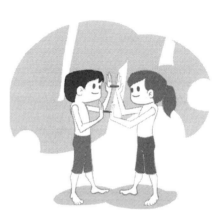

Pencils

- Once you feel comfortable moving one pencil, place the second pencil between the other two palms. So, both hands are working with a pencil in each.
- Move each hand in different directions and speeds. Can you move both pencils at once without dropping them?
- Once you feel comfortable moving two pencils in both hands sitting, stand up and walk around the room, still connected to your partner by the two pencils.
- Can you move around the room and move the pencils in unison without dropping them?
- Have fun with it! It is okay if you drop the pencils, it will happen sometimes. Pick them up, refocus, and begin again.

*Tips:

- Play around with different and more challenging ways to suspend the pencil between two partners – fingertips, toes, feet, shoulder to shoulder, back to back. Have fun!
- Teachers! Pencils provides a great mini-break in a school day to help refocus a class and build trust and teamwork among peers – with all of the advantages of meditation to boot.

Silver Thread Breathing

What is Silver Thread Breathing?

Silver Thread Breathing is a visualization technique that encourages deep breathing while offering a strong meditation component to calm and relax the body and mind.

How does it help me?

This visualization technique helps you to connect with and observe your breath. Sometimes observing your breath alone can become boring, adding the visual element of a silver thread can make it a little easier to stay present with the breath and enjoy the many benefits meditation offers.

How do I do it?

- Begin in a comfortable position, either seated or lying down.
- Gently close your eyes and begin to reflect inwardly.
- Breathe naturally, in and out through your nose.
- Slowly begin to deepen your breath by gradually increasing the length of each inhale and exhale.
- Continue breathing slowly and deeply as you shift your attention to the space between your eyebrows. The next time you breathe in – even though you are breathing in through your nose, imagine that the breath is a *silver thread entering your body at the point between your eyebrows.
- Follow the silver thread as it flows through your body all of the way to your belly button.
- As you breathe out, imagine the silver thread pulling your belly button in toward your spine, flowing back up through your body, and out the space between your eyebrows.
- Continue to breath this way for five minutes. Build on the length of time you practice each day until you can practice for 30-60 minutes.

*Tip: Be creative – you do not have to visualize a silver thread! You can imagine a beam of light, or, a favorite color washing through you. The important thing is that you follow the breath on its complete journey using the space between your eyebrows and your belly button as a guiding point to help you expand and expel the breath fully.

Dropping In

What is Dropping In?

Dropping In is a very effective exercise to quickly gain focus, or "drop in" to the present moment. It is also a very helpful tool that encourages longer meditation sessions or active meditation sessions (meaning you can do it when you are physically active, walking etc.). Utilizing the environment you are sitting or walking in as the point of focus, this exercise is especially helpful to those who may have trouble concentrating in traditional seated meditation.

How does it help me?

Present moment awareness has been known to calm the mind and quiet ruminative, obsessive or negative thought patterns, reducing feelings of distress and encouraging a positive mood. Dropping In is highly effective as a "quick fix" to refocus your attention on the present moment when you find your mind wandering.

How do I do it?

Seated or Reclined:

- Begin in a comfortable seated position, on the floor or in a chair, OR, lying comfortably on your back. Use cushions and/or blankets as needed to be as comfortable as possible.
- Gently close the eyes and take a few slow, deep breaths.
- As you begin to relax, notice any sensations around you. Observe and examine each sensation fully before moving on to the next.

Walking:

This can be practiced anywhere – walking to school or work, walking around the mall, a park or nature trail.

- Center yourself, by taking a few deep breaths in and out.
- Begin to walk very slowly and mindfully. Notice each step you take. Literally, observe in great detail as each part of your foot makes contact with the ground. Notice the pressure and sensation of each and every step you take.
- Take in your surroundings. Notice what you see, notice if it is moving or changing, what the color saturation is. Take in every detail – the color of the sky, cloud formations, and the different shades of green in each leaf.
- What other sensations can you observe? The air touching your skin? The sounds around you? Be open to different sensations and be present with each sensation as it occurs, approaching each with curiosity as though observing it for the first time.

Observation Points for Practicing Dropping In:

Physical:

- Observe what your body makes contact with: the floor, a chair, another body part etc. Notice differences between each side of the body - how it feels, pressure at contact points, temperature, clothing touching your skin etc.
- Notice where the skin makes contact with the air around you? What is the temperature? Is there a wind or breeze? Any other sensations?

Auditory:

- Observe sounds – from a buzzing mosquito to a neighbor's music. Don't attach a story to what you hear, simply observe the sounds.

Olfactory:

- Smells, observe the details of any smells.
- How do they make your nose feel? Notice your nostrils flaring, mouth watering etc. Whatever your physical responses to the smell, don't create a story about it, stay present and observe every detail of each sensation.

Visual:

- Observe the details of your surroundings. The color of the sky, changing shapes of the clouds etc.

Breath:

- Observe your breath. Be aware of the depth of the breath, which body parts move with each inhale and exhale, and how they move etc. The temperature of the air and sensations created as the breath enters and leaves your body.

*Tip:

Be careful not to allow the mind to create a "story" about the sensations you observe. For example, you might hear your neighbor's music playing. Focus solely on the sounds and vibrations of the music.

In the beginning, it will be natural for the mind to create a story such as, *"Wow, she is playing her music really loud today. I hope she turns it down when I am doing my homework later so I can concentrate. I don't even like this song, why she listens to this I have no idea…. Maybe I used to like this artist, but I like so and so now…"*. This is what the mind does all day long, without us being aware of it! One sound, one smell, one experience, can trigger an entire monologue inside our minds that can go on for minutes or even hours!

Dropping In re-trains the mind to stay in the present moment by focusing on sensations as they are and not allowing the mind to "think" about them. In the above example you would simply notice the music by the sounds and vibrations it creates without worrying or wondering about where it was coming from or who was singing.

Take Ten

What is Take Ten?

Take Ten is a breathing technique that invites relaxation and sharpens the ability to focus.

How does it help me?

Take Ten is helpful if you have a lot of mental chatter happening and you need to shift your focus. Benefits of practicing Take Ten include stress reduction and increased mental clarity. Take Ten can be practiced lying down if you are having trouble falling asleep – who says you need to count sheep? Count your breath instead!

How do I do it?

- Begin in a comfortable seated position, either in a chair with both feet on floor, or in crisscross position – (use blocks or blankets under hips and/or knees if your hips are tight). Be sure the spine is straight and the shoulders, arms and face are relaxed.
- Gently close your eyes.
- Begin to observe the breath. Do not try to control it, just let the in and out breath occur naturally.
- Begin to count each breath by saying to yourself, "I am breathing in one", "I am breathing out one", "I am breathing in two", "I am breathing out two".
- Continue to do this until you complete ten rounds of breaths. Once you reach ten, return to one and count out ten full rounds once again.
- THIS IS NOT AS EASY AS IT SOUNDS!
- Your mind will wander off and begin thinking about things. This is perfectly natural, when you notice this congratulate yourself for catching the deviation and begin counting the breath once again. BUT THERE'S A CATCH! ... You need to begin at one again.
- Have fun with this and try it often. See how far you can go before your mind tunes out.
- Can you make it to ten breaths without a mental diversion? Great! Challenge yourself by increasing the number.

Focused Breathing

What is Focused Breathing?

Focused Breathing is a relaxation technique that uses the breath as a focal point.

How does it help me?

Observing your breath is a great tool to use to help you relax when you are having trouble sleeping, it is also very effective as a meditation to help reduce feelings of stress, anxiety, or worry.

How do I do it?

- Begin in a comfortable seated position. Be sure your spine is straight and shoulders, arms and legs are relaxed.
- Close your eyes and perform a quick body scan to be sure you are comfortable and relaxed. If you feel tension anywhere do what you can to relax that area. This may be as simple as consciously relaxing a muscle, or changing the position or location of where you are sitting, or using a prop such as a pillow or blanket.
- Once you feel comfortable, close your eyes and focus on the natural rhythm of your breath. Do not force it or try to control it, simply observe how you breathe naturally.
- Keeping your eyes gently closed, begin to follow the breath's journey in great detail.
- Notice the area around the nostrils as the breath enters your body – temperature, sensation etc.
- Follow your breath through the nasal passages, to the back of the throat and down into the lungs.
- Notice your collarbones expanding.
- Follow your breath as it expands the lungs. Notice the ribs expanding too. Do they expand at the sides as well as the front and back of the torso?
- Follow the breath as you exhale, noticing the lungs relaxing as the air expels. Notice the ribs and collarbones relaxing too.
- Notice any sensations as the air exits the nostrils.
- Keep observing each step of each breath for 3-5 minutes. Be as detailed as you can.
- If your mind wanders off, simply redirect the focus to the sensations and passage of your breath and begin again.
- You may wish to add visual elements to this breathing exercise. Visualizing tension or anxiety leaving the body as you exhale. Breathing in calmness and relaxation as you inhale.
- Perhaps you can associate a color with the breath and visualize a color representing vitality as you breathe in, and a color representing relaxation as you breathe out.
- Or you can simply think of the words "calm", "relax", etc. as you breathe in and out.

Mantra

What is Mantra and how does it help me?

Meditation is a very helpful tool that can calm and sooth the body, mind and nervous system. It also relieves symptoms of stress or anxiety and improves our ability to focus. But meditating can be hard! Using a "Mantra" – a word or phrase, usually linked to the "in" and "out" breath – can help you to master and enjoy the many benefits of meditation. Think of Mantra as an anchor that keeps its ship (YOU!) firmly anchored in the present moment, rather than drifting aimlessly in an ocean of thought.

How do I do it?

- Begin in a comfortable seated position in a chair or on the floor. If sitting on the floor, prop yourself up on a pillow or bolster to ensure you can sit comfortably for longer periods.
- Gently close the eyes and turn your attention inward.
- Observe your breath as it flows in and out of your body.
- When you feel ready to begin, say your mantra inside your head as you breathe in.
- As you breathe out, repeat your mantra.
- If your mind wanders off and you catch yourself thinking about something other than your mantra, simply let go of the thoughts and refocus your attention on your breath. Observe your breath for a few rounds and then begin repeating your mantra again.

*Tips:

- Choose a mantra that works for you – one that you believe and can easily visualize.
- Focus on positives rather than negatives – for example, if you were feeling blue or sad and you were to use a mantra such as, "I am breathing in happiness", follow it with a positive like, "I am breathing out and *LETTING GO*" rather than, "I am breathing out sadness". If you're having trouble coming up with a mantra that resonates with you, use some of the following mantras as inspiration:

  "I am breathing in" … "I am breathing out"

  "I am breathing in energy" … "I am breathing out and relaxing"

  "I am breathing in the color yellow"… "I am breathing out the color green"

  "I am breathing in radiant sunshine"… "I am breathing out radiating sunshine"

  "Breathing in, I smile"…"Breathing out, I smile"

  "Breathing in, my body expands"…. "Breathing out, my body relaxes"

"Breathing in, my body feels light"… "Breathing out, my body feels lighter"

"Breathing in, I feel calm"… "Breathing out, I feel relaxed"

- The mantra you choose does not have to be an entire phrase, nor does it need to be a different word for each inhale and exhale. It can be a single word that you repeat with each "in" and "out" breath, such as:

"Happy", "Strength", "Smile", "Calm", "Relax", "Serenity", "Sunshine"

Heart Meditation

What is Heart Meditation?

Heart Meditation is exactly as it sounds, a meditation where you use your own heart and heart energy as the focal point.

How does it help me?

When learning to meditate it is helpful to have a focal point to clear your mind and truly be present. Taking time out to meditate on a daily basis improves productivity and betters your ability to focus on tasks. It is also very relaxing – think of it as a mini vacation for your body and mind. A heart meditation is a particularly nice meditation, your heart produces a lot of energy as it constantly works pumping blood throughout your body, and when you really focus on it, you can feel that energy.

How do I do it?

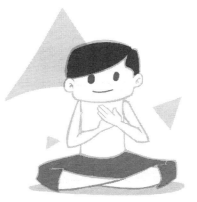

Heart Meditation

- Begin in a comfortable seated position. Spine naturally erect, both feet on the floor if seated in chair.
- Keeping your shoulders and arms relaxed, gently rest your hands on your heart area— slightly left of the center of the chest— stacking one hand on top of the other.
- Close your eyes and begin to turn your attention inward. Begin by focusing on the breath, simply observing it coming in and out.
- When you feel ready, move your attention to the area your hands are covering, your heart.
- Silently observe this area, remain seated with the eyes closed. Do not force yourself to feel anything, just sit and wait for sensations to arise.
- You may feel your heart beating, or sensations such as heat, or a vibration or buzz of energy beneath your hands. You may feel an emotion – remember the heart is not only a muscle pumping blood through our bodies, but also our center for compassion.
- If you feel a very strong energy from your heart, see if you can radiate it out to other areas of your body. That is, start with the energy you feel in the center of your chest and "grow" it, so you eventually feel that energy spreading throughout your entire body.
- Sit here for 5-10 minutes enjoying the energy from your heart.
- Gently release your hands to your lap and take several slow, deep breaths before slowly opening your eyes.

Squeeze and Release

What is Squeeze and Release?

Squeeze and Release is a relaxation technique where one systematically contracts the muscles in the body before releasing and relaxing them.

How does it help me?

Squeeze and Release relaxes the entire physical body—especially areas where you may be holding tension—preparing the body for sleep, relaxation or rest. This is a great technique to use before going to bed or before relaxing in a meditation.

How do I do it?

- Begin in a restful position lying on your back.
- Curl the toes on both feet and release – repeat several times.
- Flex and point the feet and then rotate the ankles – be sure to go in both directions.
- Resting the legs on the floor, flex the toes toward your nose – engaging the muscles in both legs. Relax and repeat several times.
- Hug the knees into the chest and squeeze them tight. Rock gently from side-to-side. Make small circles with the knees in both directions. Release and relax the legs along the floor.
- Stretch both arms overhead and point the toes away from the body, giving the entire body a stretch.
- Clench and release the fists of both hands several times. Relax the arms alongside torso and relax the feet, allowing them to fall open.
- Wrap arms across torso and give yourself a big hug, squeezing the shoulders. Release.
- Stretch the mouth open wide like a huge yawn. Release and repeat.
- Squeeze the eyes closed. Release and repeat.
- Hug the knees into the chest and squeeze them tight, tuck the chin toward the chest curling into a small ball and squeeze everything in as tight as possible – face, ears, eyes, toes – squeeze everything as tight as you can for a count of 1-2-3. And release.
- Allow the body to fully release onto the floor, imagine you are a huge puddle of water as you spread out on the floor, taking as much space as you need. Relax in this position for 5-10 minutes.

Wax Museum

What is Wax Museum?

Wax Museum is a fun relaxation technique where you start out as stiff as a wax sculpture, slowly melting in the sun down to a puddle of soft, gooey wax.

How does it help me?

Wax Museum is a meditative relaxation technique that systematically relaxes the physical body and the mind. It is helpful for anxiety, insomnia, and general physical or mental fatigue.

How do I do it?

- Begin lying on the floor, or bed/sofa.
- Stretch your arms up overhead, stretch the fingers out and point the toes. Make your body as long as you can and really S-T-R-E-T-C-H.
- Imagine you are wax sculpture – like those you would see at a wax museum.
- Release the stretch, resting arms alongside the torso, and allow the feet fall apart.
- Imagine your entire body is sculpted from wax.
- Now imagine a bright sun shining down on you. Feel its warmth all over your body.
- As your body begins to warm, imagine the wax softening.
- Beginning at the top of your head, trace your way very slowly down the entire body and imagine each part softening and melting.
- Once you visit each area of the body independently, reconnect the body as a whole and imagine it melted on the floor; one large piece of soft and gooey wax, warm from the sun. Rest here for 5-10 minutes.

Ink Bath

What is Ink Bath?

Ink Bath is a body awareness exercise that focuses on the physical body while engaging the imagination.

How does it help me?

Being fully aware and present in the body is a form of meditation. Meditation allows our minds and bodies to have a mini-break, leaving us feeling calm and relaxed and giving us the ability to be more focused and productive. Sounds like a win-win!

How do I do it?

Ink Bath can be practiced lying down or seated. Seated is good if you want to quickly refocus or take a true "mini" break; lying down is beneficial when you want to relax for a little bit longer.

- Begin in a comfortable position (lying or seated).
- Gently close the eyes and take a few deep breaths to feel centered.
- Imagine your favorite color and now imagine a bath filled with ink the exact shade of your favorite color.
- Keep your eyes closed and imagine taking bath, soaking in your favorite color.
- Imagine your entire body covered in ink, the exact shade of your favorite color.
- Now imagine the stamp or impression your body is making on the floor (or furniture) in that color.
- Slowly and carefully scan your entire body for areas that make contact with the floor (or furniture), or another part of your body, and notice what shape that area is and how much of it is making contact. What impression would it leave?
- Once you have scanned the entire body, connect it all and imagine what the entire impression would look like if you really were coated in ink. What impression would you leave on the floor or chair?
- Is it the same on both sides, or different? What shapes are there? Are they all connected or are there spaces and gaps in between? Are there heavy and dark areas and other areas with very light impressions, barely touching?
- When you feel ready, gently open your eyes. Can you still feel the areas where your body makes contact with the floor or furniture? Do you feel more aware of your body? More present?

Body Scan

What is Body Scan?

Body Scan is a relaxation technique for the mind and body.

How does it help me?

Mentally scanning the entire body by visiting one area at a time requires presence and focus, this has a deeply meditative and relaxing effect on the mind and the body. Body Scan is also a valuable tool that helps you recognize areas in the body where you hold tension, giving you the option to consciously relax these areas while practicing, as well as providing an awareness of any tension building in these areas on daily basis. When you become aware of areas or "hot spots" where you carry tension you can then consciously work to release them.

How do I do it?

- Begin in a comfortable position – preferably lying on your back. If this is not possible, sit comfortably in a chair, both feet in contact with the floor, spine naturally erect, shoulders and arms relaxed, hands resting in lap.

- Close the eyes and begin to observe the natural rhythm of your breath, following each inhale and exhale. Let go of any thoughts as you do so.

- Once you feel ready to begin, move your attention through the body. Pause at each area noting any sensation that arises and, even if that area feels relaxed, see if you can consciously relax it even more. Once that area feels completely relaxed, move on to the next point. Use the following as a guide:

  1. Top of the head – notice every detail –not just the head, but the scalp and hair.
  2. Back of the head – notice which areas contact the floor or pillow.
  3. Forehead and temples.
  4. Eyes – eyelashes and eyebrows too!
  5. Nose.
  6. Jaw – mouth, teeth and tongue too!
  7. Throat.
  8. Neck – front and back.
  9. Collarbones.
  10. Shoulders.
  11. Right upper arm, forearm, and elbow. Right hand, palm, each finger, thumb.
  12. Chest and torso.
  13. Left upper arm, forearm, and elbow. Left hand, palm, each finger, thumb.
  14. Upper back – notice which areas are in contact with the floor.
  15. Abdomen.

16. Hips - notice which areas are in contact with the floor.
17. Lower back – notice which areas are in contact with the floor.
18. Right thigh – front and back. Knee, calf and lower leg. Right foot, each toe.
19. Left thigh – front and back. Knee, calf and lower leg. Left foot, each toe.
20. Connect the whole body together. Imagine the whole body, deeply relaxed.

- Breathe and relax soaking in the sensations of a completely relaxed body. Stay here for at least 5-10 minutes, or longer if needed.

*Tips:

- If you notice tension, breathe deeply and visualize that area expanding as you inhale, and relaxing as you exhale.
- Make it fun – imagine a magic laser light glowing, warming and relaxing each area as you visit it. OR, imagine a colorful feather gently sweeping each area calming and relaxing you with light feathery strokes.

61 Point Meditation

What is 61 Point Meditation and how does it help me?

The 61 Point Meditation exercise can be practiced in two ways:

- Practiced lying down it serves as a deep relaxation exercise.
- Practiced in a seated position it serves as a concentration/focus exercise.

How do I do it?

- Refer to the attached diagram for the location of each of the 61 points on the body. (Note: It will take several practice sessions before you begin to memorize the points, enabling you to flow seamlessly through this meditation).
- Begin in a comfortable position, either seated or lying on the floor. Set yourself up to be sure you are comfortable – blankets, pillows etc.
- Relax the body as you begin to deepen the breath and settle in.
- When you feel ready to begin, shift your focus to the first point.
- Slowly move through the sequence, mentally traveling from one point in the body to the next, using one of the "61 Point Focus Tips" outlined below, all the way to the 61st point.
- Once you have visited each of the 61 points, continue to sit or lay in a relaxed state for as long as you need.

61 Point Focus Tips:

Focus: Slowly move from one point to the next, focusing all of your attention on each point as if it were the only part of your body.

Breathe: Settle on each point and remain focused on it as you breathe in and out for a count of breaths, completing the same number of breath cycles at each point. For example, count 1-5 full breath cycles at each point. Visualize the breath entering and exiting the body through each point that you are focused on.

Count: Visit each point and name it by its number as you focus on it. For example, count, "one", "two", "three"…"fifty-nine", "sixty", "sixty-one", as you visit each point.

Visualize: Visualize a color saturating each point – slowly work your way from point to point, visualizing that area of the body being bathed in a color of your choosing. For example, blue is a very calming color. It may also be helpful to visualize a shape, such as a blue star or circle pulsing at each point.

*Tip: Create a recording of the points, or have somebody read them to you so that you can fully engage in the exercise without referring to the chart.

1. Center of forehead
2. Base of front of neck
3. Right shoulder
4. Right elbow
5. Right wrist
6. Right thumb
7. Right index finger
8. Right middle finger
9. Right ring finger
10. Right little finger
11. Right wrist
12. Right elbow
13. Right shoulder
14. Base of front of neck
15. Left shoulder
16. Left elbow
17. Left wrist
18. Left thumb
19. Left index finger
20. Left middle finger
21. Left ring finger
22. Left little finger
23. Left wrist
24. Left elbow
25. Left shoulder
26. Base of front of neck
27. Center of chest
28. Right side of chest
29. Center of chest
30. Left side of chest
31. Center of chest
32. Belly button
33. Lower belly
34. Right hip
35. Right knee
36. Right ankle
37. Right big toe
38. Right second toe
39. Right third toe
40. Right fourth toe
41. Right little toe
42. Right Ankle
43. Right knee
44. Right hip
45. Lower belly
46. Left hip
47. Left knee
48. Left ankle
49. Left big toe
50. Left second toe
51. Left third toe
52. Left fourth toe
53. Left little toe
54. Left ankle
55. Left knee
56. Left hip
57. Lower belly
58. Belly button
59. Center of chest
60. Base of front of neck
61. Center of forehead

61 Point Meditation

Magic Carpet Ride

What is Magic Carpet Ride?

Magic Carpet Ride is a guided relaxation technique often used in kid's yoga classes, but this does not mean it is just for kids! Adults and teens also enjoy–and *benefit* from— the freedom of choosing and imagining a journey to a special place of their own.

How does it help me?

Magic Carpet Ride gives you the power to choose, dream, imagine, escape and let go. It is very relaxing and, since you are creating the journey in your mind, you are free to keep it to yourself or share it with others once you finish. It is a great exercise that provides a safe haven you can visit anytime you feel the need to take a break from your every day life.

How do I do it?

- Begin in a comfortable resting position, preferably on your back. (Can be seated if lying down is uncomfortable for any reason).

- Lights should be turned down and blankets and pillows used to help you be as relaxed and comfortable as possible.

- Gently close the eyes and leave them closed for the duration of this exercise.

- Take a few deep breaths as you scan your body from head to toe to be sure it is relaxed and floppy.

- Imagine the surface beneath you is a beautiful magic carpet. Imagine every detail: What color is it? Does it have any patterns or embellishments? What fabric it is made from? What texture is it? This is YOUR magic carpet, so make it anything you want.

- Feel your beautiful magic carpet beneath you, holding you, supporting you and keeping you safe. Notice as the magic carpet begins to gently lift you off the floor, light as a feather yet fully supported, it gently lifts you up and out of the room.

- Feel the wind gently caress your face and body as your magic carpet slowly drifts up over the city where you began this journey. Drifting past the clouds, your magic carpet lifts you up, higher and higher, over the treetops. Listen to the birds in the trees chirping hello to you as you float by.

- Passing by the clouds, you could reach out and touch their billowy softness they are so near. Feel the wind gently caress you, the soft clouds touching you as you float by, fully supported, safe and secure on your beautiful magic carpet. Drifting toward your very special, magic place – it can be anywhere: a park, the beach, a forest, another city or country, another planet, or a special magical land, anywhere that you want to go that feels special to you! Your magic carpet has the ability to travel anywhere you can imagine, just picture it in your mind and it will take you there.

- Feel the wind caress your face as your magic carpet gently lowers you down to your special, magic place. Light as a feather, safe and secure, gently placing you in your special magic place.

- Notice how it feels to be in your special magic place, notice the sounds around you... What do you hear? …. Notice the smells in your special magic place… What does it smell like? …. Notice who is here with you in your special magic place? ... You are safe, secure and happy, enjoying your very own special place. Knowing you can come here anytime you like… it belongs to you.

- Stay as long as you like, enjoying all of the sensations of being here. When you are ready to return, take one last look around and know that you can come back anytime. Wave goodbye to your special place, to all of the people or animals or creatures there, and know you can visit them again anytime you like.

- Feel your magic carpet gently lift you up, floating up ever so slowly to the sky. Touch the soft fluffy clouds as you drift by and feel the breeze touch your skin as your magic carpet makes its way back to where you began this journey. Feel the warm sun shining on your face, as you float in the sky, ever so safely, on your beautiful magic carpet. Hear the birds chirping, "Hello! Welcome back!" as you float on down over the treetops and into your city and then, finally, softly landing back where you began.

- Rest here as long as you like, taking in all of the sensations and remembering all of the details of your amazing journey.

- Once you feel ready, slowly sit up and, if you like, you can share your experience with a friend or simply write a journal entry or draw a picture about your adventure.

*Tip:

Teachers, when guiding a group or class, gently suggest students imagine and answer your questions in their minds rather than speaking aloud.

You may need to keep gently reminding them, or pose the question or suggestion to preface this. Such as, "Now inside your mind, imagine what color you magic carpet is"… or, "Remember this is your secret special place, so keep it a secret in your mind as you land your magic carpet in your special place."

The BIG Chillax

What is the BIG Chillax?

The BIG Chillax is exactly as it sounds, a BIG moment to simply do nothing other than chill and relax – giving your body and mind the BIG rest it deserves.

How does it help me?

Imagine leaving your computer or iPod on all day, every day – it would eventually lose its charge and not work at all. Well, your mind and body are no different! With our bodies constantly on the go physically, our mind often chats away incessantly too – creating stories, planning, remembering etc. Turning everything off and giving yourself a little recharge will not only make you feel good but will give you more energy to do the things you love and do them well.

How do I do it?

- Begin in a comfortable position lying on the floor.
- Prop a pillow under the knees to release any pressure from the lower back and a pillow under the head for comfort. The body temperature drops when you relax so keep a blanket close by in case you need it.
- Allow the feet to fall apart and the arms to rest alongside the torso with the palms facing up. Gently close your eyes and take a few deep inhales and exhales before allowing the breath to fall into its natural rhythm.
- Let go. Allow the physical body to " let go", and be fully supported by the floor and pillows. Allow the mind to "let go" releasing any thoughts – this part will not be easy! The mind will always want to "think", "chat", "talk" – it is constantly running a "commentary" – the trick here, is to let it do its thing without encouraging it by attaching to any of those thoughts. If you find yourself trailing along with the mind on a long commentary, simply stop and detach yourself from it. Do this each time the mind tries to get your attention. Let it go.
- The aim of The BIG Chillax is to stop doing and simply "be". Be calm. Be still. Be relaxed. Let go. Do nothing. Chill. Relax. Chillax.
- Remain in this relaxed state for 10-30 minutes. When it is time to finish do so slowly. Gently rouse the mind and body by deepening your breath, slowly move the tongue around in the mouth. Gently wiggle fingers and toes and then roll wrists and ankles.
- When you feel ready, draw the knees in toward your chest and roll onto one side into a fetal position. Rest here for a moment before gently using your arms to press yourself up in to a comfortable seated position.
- Sit with the eyes closed for a few moments and enjoy the sensations of feeling relaxed.

*Tip: To really enjoy the benefits of the BIG Chillax be sure to make yourself as comfortable as possible - dim the lights, close the shades, play soothing music and use pillows, blankets and eye pillows.

Ocean Drift

What is Ocean Drift?

Ocean Drift is an auditory meditation technique that relaxes the mind and body.

What do I need?

- Comfortable place to lie still and relax.
- *Ocean sounds track (Downloadable from iTunes – See recommendations below)
- Sound system to play track.
- Pillows, blankets, bolsters as needed for comfort.

How do I do it?

- Set up sound system to "loop" ocean sounds track for as long as you would like to enjoy this meditation/relaxation exercise.
- Begin to play track and turn the lights off or down before getting comfortable.
- Lie down on your back and set yourself up with any props necessary to be comfortable – pillows, blankets etc.
- Take several deep breaths as your body releases and relaxes onto the floor, allow the mind to let go of any thoughts as you settle in and relax.
- Let the body go completely, allowing the floor to fully support it.
- Shift your attention to the sounds filling the room.
- Allow the waves to wash over you. Each wave bringing a new and deeper sense of relaxation to your body and mind. Releasing any tension with each receding wave. Allow the ocean to ebb and flow, maintaining a focus on the sounds.
- Once the Ocean meditation is over, rest a little longer without the music enjoying the benefits of this exercise before slowly sitting up.

*Tip: Ocean sound tracks are available from iTunes. You may also find some on relaxation CD's available at local music stores, health food stores, or department stores such as Walmart or Target. Ocean sounds may be substituted for any track you find soothing and relaxing – forest sounds, birds, water etc.

Recommendations:

Ocean Waves Solo - A Meditative Journey, Natalie Maisel – www.yogadownload.com

Ocean Waves 1 – Sounds For Life – iTunes

Ocean Sounds – New Born Baby Lullabies – iTunes

Sleeping Mouse

What is Sleeping Mouse?

Sleeping Mouse is a restorative body posture, meaning there is no physical effort required. Also known as child's pose or rock pose, Sleeping Mouse is a resting posture that allows the body and mind to relax.

How does it help me?

Sleeping Mouse releases tension in the back, shoulders and chest while gently lengthening and stretching the spine, as well as stretching the hips, thighs and ankles. It alleviates stress and anxiety, calming the mind and body and is highly recommended if you feel dizzy or fatigued.

How do I do it?

- Come to your knees and sit back onto your heels.
- Slowly fold the upper body forward so that your torso rests on your thighs.
- Stack your fists and rest your forehead on them. Breathe.
- Gently move your fists and allow your forehead to rest on the floor.
- Rest your arms back along side your torso and legs, with the palms facing up. Breathe deeply and rest here for as long as your like.
- To move out of Sleeping Mouse. Slowly stretch your arms back in front of you on the floor and walk the hands in toward the body as you rise to seated position.

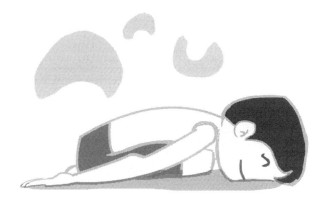

Sleeping Mouse

*Tip: If you experience pain in your knees, or you have a knee injury, simply lie on your back and hug your knees in toward your chest. Keep your head and shoulders resting on the floor and close your eyes. Breathe slowly.

Rainbow, Rainbow Meditation

What is Rainbow, Rainbow Meditation?

Rainbow, Rainbow Meditation is a visualization technique that draws on nature and color therapy to help you feel relaxed, vibrant and confident.

How does it help me?

Color therapy is based on the theory that colors can trigger certain psychological or emotional states. For example, Blue is known to be calming, while Yellow is known to be energizing. As you relax in your Rainbow, Rainbow Meditation, you will be guided to visualize the different colors of the rainbow and the positive mind states each color represents. After this meditation you should feel radiant and fabulous... just like a rainbow!

How do I do it?

- Begin in a comfortable position lying on the floor.
- Prop a pillow under the knees to release any pressure on the low back and a pillow under the head for comfort. Body temperature drops when you relax, so keep a blanket close by in case you need it.
- Allow the feet to fall apart and the arms to rest alongside the torso, with the palms facing up. Gently close your eyes and take a few deeply relaxing inhales and exhales before allowing the breath to fall into its natural rhythm.
- Imagine floating on a soft billowy cloud, light as feather yet fully supported.
- Imagine the arc of beautiful rainbow spreading above you. Beginning at your toes and arcing up over your body to your head.
- Imagine as each color baths you from toes to your head, and back again. Connecting your whole body beneath the image of a rainbow:

  RED: POWERFUL and STRONG

  ORANGE: JOYFUL and CREATIVE

  YELLOW: SUNNY and CONFIDENT

  GREEN: KIND and LOVING

  BLUE: CALM and HONEST

  INDIGO: CLEVER and INTUITIVE

  VIOLET: LOYAL and WISE

- Take your time to truly feel and experience each color before moving on the next.
- Relax and rest under your completed rainbow, soaking in its vibrant energy for as long as you like.

Crocodile

What is Crocodile?

Crocodile is a restorative body posture that uses props rather than muscle engagement to support the body and maintain the posture, allowing the body to relax fully.

How does it help me?

Crocodile is a very grounding posture, meaning the body and mind will feel anchored and connected to the present moment rather than scattered and/or anxious. It is very calming and relaxing.

What do I need?

- A bolster (or folded up blanket or pillow)
- A yoga block*

How do I do it?

- Lie face down on your belly, placing yoga bolster (or folded blanket) under your ribcage.
- Place a yoga block under your forehead.
- Relax your arms and legs completely, allowing the body to be fully supported by the props and the floor.
- Breathe deeply, feeling the belly expand and release against the floor.
- Allow yourself to be heavy, imagine sinking deeper into the floor with each exhale.
- Stay in this deeply relaxing posture for 5-10 minutes.

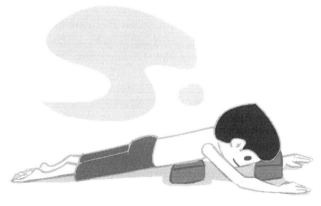

Crocodile

*Tip: If you do not have a block you can stack your hands or fists on top of one another and rest your forehead on the top hand/fist.

About the Author

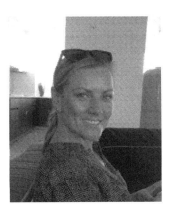

Lisa Roberts has been involved in the pediatric wellness field since 2006. As the first complementary therapist to work from the inception of a pediatric wellness program for oncology patients and their families/caregivers at New York University's Hassenfeld Center for Cancer and Blood Disorders, Lisa offered weekly Reiki sessions in the clinic, in addition to workshops for families and staff to learn Reiki during weekends. The program has since grown to offer additional wellness modalities.

In 2008, following a move to Saint Louis MO, she volunteered at a major children's hospital to continue her work offering wellness techniques to staff. Launching YoYo Yoga Therapy, a private yoga therapy practice for kids aged 1 to 101, in 2011, Lisa was hired as an independent contractor as the hospital's first yoga instructor, responsible for creating the curriculum and teaching yoga to patients, patient siblings, and staff. She has been invited to speak about the benefits of wellness, complementary therapies and yoga to support groups in addition to leading yoga and meditation classes at summer camps for patients and a drop in center for at risk youth.

When not teaching or practicing yoga, Lisa works as a freelance editor and writer. Passionate about travel, especially to her homeland Australia, she enjoys getaways with her husband Michael, as well as hanging out in Saint Louis with their grandchildren, Audrey, Noah and Jonah, beloved family and friends, and one very spoiled kitty-cat called Anabella.

Made in the USA
Lexington, KY
16 September 2014